Special Delivery

An Obstetrician's Honest Account of a
Forty-Year Career in a Changing Healthcare Environment

KENNETH J. MOISE, JR. M.D.

Special Delivery
An Obstetrician's Honest Account of a Forty-Year Career in a Changing Healthcare Environment
©2023, Kenneth J. Moise, Jr. M.D.

Cover photo: Dr. Moise performs an ultrasound on his second-
born daughter and his yet undelivered third grandchild.

My goal for this book is to portray a true account of the events that have occurred in my academic
career. This of course is limited to my memory of these events.
The names of the patients and physicians have been altered to protect their privacy.
The content is not meant to be malicious or harmful to any individual or institution.
Instead, the intent is to portray a level of transparency for the public at large.

The opinions expressed within are solely that of the author and do not reflect the
views and policies of Dell Medical School—University of Texas at Austin.

ISBN 978-1-66788-988-7
ISBN eBook 978-1-66788-989-4

TABLE OF CONTENTS

Dedication

I would like to dedicate this book to the many physician mentors that have influenced my journey in medicine. Many are retired while some are deceased. My experiences with them remain forever etched in my memory.

I would be remiss if I did not acknowledge my wife, Karen. She has given me three amazing daughters. Throughout my career, she has been my confidant and my biggest supporter. She has truly been my rock.

1

Prologue

The little black box on my belt squealed with an ear-piercing sound—
"beep, beep, beep." I looked down at its LED display—my secretary
paging me. I grabbed the desk phone nearby and called my office.
"There is a patient on the phone from Florida that would like to talk
with you," she said.

"Ok, can you go ahead and connect me," I responded.

"Dr. Moise, I know you are busy but could I talk with you about
my high-risk pregnancy?" came the voice over the line.

"Sure, go ahead," I responded.

"My name is Kathy and I want to see if you will take care of me.
I been looking up medical articles in the library and I think you are
considered an expert on the condition I have," she said.

"Tell me your story," I replied. Kathy's blood type was Rh negative. In her first pregnancy, she had delivered a little girl, but at the
time of the delivery, her obstetrician determined that she had *Rh anti-*

bodies in her bloodstream. The usual injection given to most Rh-negative patients to prevent these antibodies from forming would no longer work. In her next pregnancy, Kathy's *antibody titer* (a measure of the amount of antibody in her bloodstream) turned out to be very high. But unfortunately, her doctor did not follow her pregnancy that closely.

"One day at around six months into my pregnancy, my baby boy stopped moving," she told me. "I called my Ob's office and they told me to come in right away. I watched anxiously as the technician poured gel on my belly and placed the ultrasound probe to find my baby's heartbeat. She searched in vain for several minutes. Then she informed me that she needed to get the doctor. Several anxious minutes went by. I just knew something was wrong. My Ob doc came into the room. Without saying a word, he placed the ultrasound on my pregnant belly and again began to look around. After a few moments he confirmed by biggest fear – my baby boy's heart had stopped."

Kathy went on with her story, "They sent me to the emergency room. After about two hours of waiting in the exam room, an emergency room doctor came in. He did another ultrasound to confirm there was no heartbeat. He then called the on-call obstetrician who told him I should see my primary OB in the morning. By this time my husband had arrived and he was getting angry. We decided to drive to another hospital ER but the answers there were the same – the ER could do nothing and the on-call OB did not want to take care of me."

Kathy paused for a moment on the phone call to collect her thoughts, "Just before I was discharged for the second time, a nurse came by and told me she had called one of the OB physicians she knew. She told me that he would take care of me. We began the induction of labor later that night. Our little boy was born six hours later. I gazed at him and noted how perfect and peaceful he looked wrapped in this blue birthing blanket. We decided to name him Hope."

Hemolytic disease of the fetus/newborn is the result of a difference in blood types between a pregnant woman (who is Rh negative) and her unborn child (who is Rh positive due to genes inherited from its father). In some situations, red blood cells from the fetus escape into the woman's blood stream, are recognized as foreign to her and antibodies are formed. In most cases, this immune reaction can be prevented by giving the Rh-negative pregnant patient a special injection (called *Rhesus immune globulin*) in the seventh month of pregnancy and again at the time of delivery. But sometimes this fails, and Rh antibodies form in the patient. If she carries a Rh-positive fetus in her next pregnancy, the antibodies can cross through the placenta and attack the fetal red blood cells. This can then cause severe *anemia* (low blood count) in the fetus and even death. This is called *hemolytic disease of the fetus/newborn*.

"I'm now eight weeks pregnant, Dr. Moise," Kathy said. "I am so scared. Could this happen to me again? I can't go through losing another baby."

"I understand, Kathy," I responded. "Let's see what we can do. I want you to see Dr. Schneider, a *Maternal-Fetal Medicine specialist* (a board-certified subspecialist in high-risk obstetrics), who has an office near where you live. He will do ultrasounds every week and if he thinks the baby is getting into trouble, he will refer you to me if you need special treatments."

Six months into the pregnancy, Kathy called back. Through tears, she told me, "They say my baby has hydrops and could die any day. This can't be happening!"

"I want you to catch the next flight here," I told her. Kathy arrived the next morning and an ultrasound indeed revealed that her unborn daughter was near death due to severe anemia. Later that same afternoon, we performed an emergency *intrauterine transfusion*—we used ultrasound to guide a needle into the fetal umbilical cord and give life-saving Rh-negative red blood cells.

The following day, the baby's condition showed marked improved on the ultrasound. Thanksgiving was two days away. Kathy was a fireman in Florida and a one-way return plane ticket before the upcoming holiday was more than she could afford. Karen, my wife, was one of our nurse coordinators at our Fetal Center. She called the local *Ronald McDonald House*. Pretty much every pediatric hospital in our country has one of these special temporary residences for families with sick pediatric patients.

"I know this is unusual, but I have a pregnant woman with a very sick baby on board that has come all the way from Florida for treatment," Karen said. "Is there any way you could bend the rules a bit and let her stay with you through Thanksgiving?" They acquiesced. But there would be no family Thanksgiving dinner for Kathy.

"You must come to our house for Thanksgiving," Karen told her. "Ken will pick you up from the Ronald McDonald House."

There were about fifteen folks at our dinner table for the holiday meal the next day. Dr. Stan James, my partner, happened to pull up a chair next to Kathy. "I think I've met you before somewhere," he said turning to her.

"That's right," she replied. "I was lying on the operating room table two days ago when you were assisting Dr. Moise. I came here to give thanks for the wonderful things you'll do."

I have spent my entire career of four decades in academic medicine. When most patients seek medical care, they see a physician in private practice. For the most part, the mission of these physicians is to care for patients. Academic physicians are affiliated with one of the 141 accredited medical schools in the USA. Their mission is threefold: research, teaching, and clinical care. This book chronicles my journey from undergraduate education to medical school to my role as a tenured full professor at several major medical universities. In it, I attempt to educate the reader on how our medical schools improve our country's heath care by aiding in the discovery of new treatments for disease. Academic physicians also serve to train the next generation of physicians. And then, we take care of patients. Often, this involves supervising residents in training; sometimes we care for our own patients.

Medicine is a unique profession. Because you wear a white coat or a pair of scrubs, a patient entrusts you with their innermost secrets. They put their lives (and in the case of the pregnant women I have cared for, their unborn baby's life) in the hands of a perfect stranger after little more than a handshake greeting. It is truly a privilege to engender this degree of trust even in the most trying of times. It is not to be taken lightly.

I have seen significant changes in health care over the past four decades. Some are good and some have led to increased physician burnout and patient dissatisfaction. The careful history and physical examination were once the centerpiece of the patient interaction. The patient was asked to tell you her story in her own words followed by a physical examination–a laying of the hands to decipher any signs of disease. These steps were essential to the art of medicine. Today, however, sophisticated blood tests and advanced imaging procedures are the norm to make a diagnosis. Indeed, the art of medicine has now being replaced by the science of medicine. Patient information is now entered into the *electronic medical record* (*EMR*) on a computer screen—a further distraction from interacting directly with our patients.

Academic medicine has changed too. Shrinking monies in health care have led many medical schools to have their faculty focus on clinical productivity often to the detriment of clinical research and teaching. It is my sincere hope that the reader will be afforded the opportunity to follow my journey from first learning to do clinical research to later mentoring physician trainees. Insights into the politics of medicine are divulged through my roles at multiple academic institutions where I have worked in my career.

Physicians learn their trade through patient experience. Throughout the book, I have chosen to recount some of the patient anecdotes that remain permanently etched in my memory. The names of the patients and the physicians have been changed to protect anonymity. In the final chapters, I take the reader through a journal in health care as seen through my eyes as a physician—first as a patient and then as a caregiver and an advocate for my wife.

It is my sincere hope that you will find this memoir both entertaining and enlightening. The average citizen is naïve to many of the inner sanctums of health care. However, one of the goals in my writing this book is to impart a little more knowledge of the workings and the politics of academic medicine as well as medicine in general. At times, the prose may be perceived as somewhat frank. The opinions expressed are solely mine and are not meant in any way to be offensive to the reader or to the medical profession as a whole.

2

So, You Want To Be a Doctor?

I didn't grow up wanting to be a physician. I am a product of education by the Jesuit order. My high school bragged that all of its graduates went on to college. I developed a love for writing and even enrolled in a college-level course during my senior year. My dad was the first member of his family to graduate from college. His expectation was that the oldest of his five sons would do the same, setting an example for the younger siblings. But, in my last year of high school, I was conflicted as to my future path in life. An aptitude test to look for guidance to a future career pointed me to a degree in journalism—a career that did not please my father's idea of a stable career path. In high school, I had only taken courses in chemistry and physics and had missed the opportunity for exposure to biology. As I headed to college, I decided to see if I had any interest in the biologic sciences.

The auditorium room was filled with over a thousand eager freshman college students. The deans of the various colleges sat at a long table at the front of the room.

The dean of engineering was the first to speak. "All engineering majors, please exit the side entrance of the auditorium and report to room 200." About fifty students left their seats and exited.

The dean of education spoke next. "All education majors, please follow me to room 300." One hundred and fifty students left. And so it went dean after dean until only the Dean of Arts and Sciences remained at the head of the room.

He then announced, "So you are the pre-med group." The auditorium remained almost half full! I knew that there were only three medical schools in my state that accepted a total of approximately 300 new medical students each year. I looked around the auditorium and knew that this was going to be a competition!

In earlier times, students interested in becoming a physician would enroll in a university to take *pre-med* courses—biology, chemistry, mathematics, etc. They would apply to medical school early in the third year of college and if accepted would begin their medical school training the following year. After completing their first year of medical school, they would return to the university to receive their *Bachelor of Science* degree. By the time I was interested in becoming a physician, virtually all medical schools required a four-year undergraduate degree as a pre-requisite. Most of us sought a degree in a life science—biology, chemistry, etc. However today, many medical schools are looking for a more well-rounded individual. Only about two-thirds of today's medical students get a degree in a biology-related field[1]. Others major in disciplines like English literature or Spanish and take the standard medical school pre-requisites such as biology and organic chemistry. Extracurricular activities are valued. When I look at medical school applications today, I am amazed. Many applicants have taken a year off to do mission work in Africa or Central America. In my day, I worked every summer to help pay for my educational expenses. Times were different then. I think it would probably be a challenge for me to be accepted to medical school today.

Comparative anatomy with Professor Clare was considered the true test for the pre-med student at my university. After all, this professor had taught the class for almost forty years and he wrote the textbook and the lab manual we would use. Rumor was that an "A" in comparative anatomy was almost a guaranteed admission to the state medical school. So, I set out in the fall semester of my second year in college to achieve that goal. I had attended a college prep high school and had tested out of several university courses receiving advanced credit for twelve semester hours. This allowed me to schedule a "light semester" of twelve hours (a typical pre-med semester would be fifteen to eighteen hours to complete the one hundred twenty total hours need for a *Bachelor of Science* degree in four years). So when I went to the registration area at the basketball auditorium at the start of the semester, I only pulled IBM computer cards to schedule comparative anatomy (four hours), organic chemistry (three hours), advanced Spanish (three hours) and tennis (two hours). What I could not figure out is why I would only get four hours of credit for comparative anatomy. My schedule read—one-hour lecture on Monday, Wednesday, and Friday and an additional lab for one and one-half hours on Tuesday and Thursday. Now to my calculation that was six hours of work for four hours of credit. Go figure!

On the first day of class this stocky, five-foot-tall professor with wire-rimmed glasses walked in. "I will only give out five "A's" to this class of 150 students," he stated. "I have a proven way of grading each of your three lecture tests and your two lab exams. There will ONLY be five A's. At the end of the year, just before the final exam, I will offer a make-up test that will look just like the final examination. If you decide to take that test, you can use the grade to replace one of your earlier exams." *No problem*, I thought, I will be one of the five A's.

I had decided to go to the state university late in my senior year of high school after turning down a scholarship at a smaller state university. As a result, my dormitory assignment was the *stadium*. Now the stadium dormitory was built early in the school's history when the governor at the time wanted to build a large football stadium for his lead state university. The state budget was tight so the legislature would not approve of such an extravagant expenditure. Solution: build a student dormitory under the stands in the shape of an oval. Put a football field inside the oval. Freshman dormitory and football stadium approved! Today the stadium dormitories are no longer used by students; the football stadium has undergone the addition of multiple upper desks and is one the largest in the south.

Tim was my roommate that semester. He was a likeable fellow from a small town in the northern part of the state. His life's dream was to go to medical school but coming from a public high school, he really had never been challenged to develop study habits to allow for the transition to a large state university. Tim took comparative anatomy with me. It came time for the first lecture exam. I had outlined virtually every chapter with a hi-lighter—that see-through marker that forces you to read everything twice—the first read followed by the speed read a second time when you are marking the sentence. One would think that you would highlight only the important things but in fact most of the chapters in my textbook were all in yellow. Tim failed the first test. I made a "high B." I was devastated. Were my dreams for medical school over? What had I missed? All of the assigned chapters were highlighted. I had even copied my class lectures notes over each night after that day's lecture. Professor Clare had pulled a fast one—he had asked questions from the glossary in the back of the book! I vowed never again to get caught unprepared. I did the calculations for the grading curve Dr. Clare had proposed on the first day—I could achieve an "A" but only if all of my other exam scores were "A's". The time arrived for the first lab practical exam—we had completed the dissection and studied the anatomy of a shark. Not too complicated. Easy enough—an "A". Tim made a "C." Several weeks passed and I knew Dr. Clare would not catch me off guard this time.

It was now time for the second lecture exam. I studied for weeks even using a different colored highlighter for the second section of the book (and the glossary). It was my practice before these exams to briefly go over my notes the night before the test and then to go to bed early. After all I had been preparing for weeks and what else could I memorize. Tim didn't study that way. He would party most nights and then the night before the exam he would "pull an all-nighter" and "cram." This usually meant lots of coffee and a trip to the local pharmacy for *No-Doz*—caffeine pills equivalent to about five cups of coffee.

"Heh, can I borrow your alarm clock tonight so I can get up early to finish cramming?" Tim asked.

"Sure, but be sure to set it for me for seven so I can have time to get breakfast and get to the exam at eight," I responded.

Off to sleep I went. I awoke the next morning with the sun streaming through the window into my eyes. One glance at the clock—9 a.m. Oh god! I had slept through my test! I quickly dressed and headed straight to Professor Clare's office and parked myself on the floor outside his door. He soon returned with a large pile of test papers under his arm.

"Dr. Clare I am one of your students in comparative anatomy and I accidentally slept through this morning's test," I said. "I have not spoken to anyone about the exam and have come straight here. Is there any way I can take this exam in your office?"

"Well son," he said looking over the top of his gold rimmed glasses, "seems like you will get a zero on today's exam. There is always the makeup exam at the end of the semester. You can use that grade to replace the exam you missed." I was devastated—my dreams of medical school seemed over.

I later figured out that Tim had set my alarm for 5 a.m. and awakened to "cram" for a few more hours before the exam. He then headed out to breakfast without resetting the alarm clock. About fifteen minutes into the exam, he realized his roommate was conspicuously absent. I never saw Tim again that semester. I later learned when the grades were posted that he had failed the exam. He left school with dashed dreams of going to medical school.

When I finally did return to my dorm room after speaking with Dr. Clare, I had decided to quit college. Perhaps I would go back to being a framing carpenter—a summer job in which I had become quite proficient during my later high school summers. I grabbed my pillow case and threw in a razor, a comb, and a toothbrush and headed home. My parents were quite surprised to see me appear at the front door. I was their firstborn of five sons who had always excelled in school. I was destined to be the first physician in the family.

My dad and I had many long discussions over the ensuing weekend. "You have never failed before and I know how much you wanted to do well in this course," he said. "But I still have faith in you that you can turn this around."

Sunday night I decided to head back to the university to give it a go. Making an "A" in comparative anatomy became my life's mission. I dropped down to eight semester hours (the minimum number to still be called a full-time student who could live on campus). Getting an "A" on my next lecture test and lab practical gave me confidence that I might still have hope.

The final lab dissection involved the cat as a specimen. The cats were provided by the university and were obtained from a scientific supply house. They came nicely injected with blue latex rubber in their veins and red latex rubber injected in the arteries. I soon came to learn that like many of the anatomical dissections in my future education, it would be virtually impossible to match the pace of the lab manual with the limited time assigned to the laboratory periods. Worse, we were not allowed to come to the lab to work after hours. Solution: we found our own scientific supply house and three members of our study group chipped in to buy our own injected cat. We weren't allowed to have refrigerators in our dorm rooms (something about the wiring being outdated in the stadium dorms). Bill, my lab partner, offered to store the cat in his refrigerator at his apartment since he lived in married student housing. Needless to say, Amy, his wife, was not pleased when the study group would all show up at their tiny apartment to undertake dissections on their kitchen table.

The final week of the semester rolled around. The final lab practical was Friday morning on the cat anatomy, the make-up final lecture exam was Friday night, and the regular lecture final exam was scheduled for Monday morning. A long weekend of testing! I "aced" the practical in the morning and treated myself to a big lunch as the student union. When I entered the exam room that night for the make-up lecture exam, there were about fifty students from the comparative anatomy class who had decided to take the exam as a replacement grade for one of their previous exams. Needless to say, I was the only student who need to replace a "zero" score.

Professor Clare stood with the pile of exam papers at the front of the room. "If you decide that you do not want this exam to count, please bring it up to the front and I will tear it up," he instructed.

For the next ninety minutes, my concentration was periodically interrupted by the sound of shredding paper. When I looked up at the end of the exam period, ten of us remained in the room and turned in our exams. I would not know my grade on the make-up exam until later, but I thought I had done well.

The rest of the weekend passed slowly as I reviewed all of my class notes and the entire Clare text in preparation for the final exam. The alarm clock woke me up on time for the final exam on Monday morning. I knew halfway through that I was going to make the grade.

On the way back to my dorm I felt a sense of relief and exhilaration. In the classic book *The House of God*, Dr. Roy Bash finishes his tumultuous intern year and celebrates by throwing his medical bag across the parking lot of the hospital as he exits for the last time. In a similar act of catharsis, I grabbed my copy of Professor Clare's text and threw it the length of the dormitory hall. I had given it my best shot. Tuesday came—I was given the only "A" on the makeup exam. "A's" on the final practical and final exam—an "A" in the course. I had succeeded! I still have my comparative anatomy text on my bookshelf with a few other texts I keep from my early years in education. I leaf through it every now and then to remember the yellow, pink, and blue highlighter colors.

The rest of my pre-med semesters were nowhere as challenging both emotionally or academically. My intended degree was a *Bachelor of Science in Zoology*, not that I was planning to care for animals in a caged setting. Our state university offered this degree instead of the usual degree most pre-med majors signed up for, biology. The Zoology degree enabled the pre-med students to take some less strenuous coursework to "pad" their schedule. We were also required to take at least one natural zoology class. And so it was that it came time in the first semester of my junior year that I had to choose between *ornithology* (the study of birds) and *ichthyology* (the study of fish). Rumor among the pre-med group was that *ichthyology* was the easier choice.

I showed up for the first lecture not knowing want to expect. Three hours of straight lecture on Monday nights every week—how could this be possible? And yet, Professor Green made this a wonderful experience with his many stories of the evolution of fish interspersed with tales of his own fishing trips around the world. Of course, there was the pre-requisite laboratory that accompanied all biology courses. There were two "fishing trips" that were scheduled; we had to attend only one of these. The first involved a visit to the nearby coastal town for some beach rod and reel fishing. The second involved a day trip up the interstate highway to "seine" a "borrow pit." This sounded interesting, so I signed up for the second option. Clearly this turned out to be the better choice.

On the day of the trip, we all showed up at a parking lot at the university. We rode in two vans for about an hour and then pulled over to the shoulder of the interstate highway in the middle of nowhere. We grabbed the coolers and two sets of large nets. Trudging through the woods we came to the "borrow pit." As it turned out, this small pond of murky water was used for fill by construction crews to build up the road base for the nearby highway. We were then instructed by the accompanying grad students who were supervising the operation to roll out the nets. *Seining* it turns out is to drag a net through a body of water using the poles attached to either end. One then pulls the net through the center of the pond and then over to the shore to see what fish (and other debris) have been caught. Much to our surprise, the first pass yielded more fish than the nets of the disciples in the sea of Galilee. Most were carp but there were a variety of smaller species.

Several of us got excited about the number of carp that filled our nets.

"Can we take these back to our dorm for a fish fry?" we asked.

"Sure," said one of the grad students. "But do you know how to cook them; it is very important?"

"Barbecue or fry in oil?" I asked.

"Nope. Nail them to a board and smoke them for several hours," he responded. Then take them off the board, throw them away and eat the board." Clearly, carp were the bottom feeders of the pond and were to be returned to their native habitat. After harvesting one or two carp as "native" fish, we went on to collect as many other species as possible. All were added to the coolers. Two more passes of the seine and the coolers contained some fifty or more different types of fish.

The following week, we returned to the lab. On all the desks were fifty different jars of formaldehyde, each containing an individual species of fish.

The zoology graduate student overseeing our lab provided us with instruction. "Open your lab manuals," he said. You will be required to identify the genus and species of each of these fish. Your final practical will be on the very fish that you caught".

If only we had known—we would not have been so enthusiastic in our catch! How would it be possible remember all of these fish – they all looked alike. And how could we memorize the Latin genus and species to identify each? Was this the *crip* (easy) course I had heard about? But wait, then our instructor had let us in on the real secret—these were the SAME fish that we would be tested on for our practical exam. But how many extra hours would have to be spent in the lab at night to memorize all of this?

Then an epiphany—take photos of all the fish in the jars with the identifying labels on them! And so it was that once the class had successfully identified all of our "catch," I entered the lab one night with my Kodak camera loaded with slide film and carefully photographed all fifty fish. Our study group of course made sure that the slides were all developed and turned out to be of decent quality. The weekend before the final practical, we met and reviewed the slides for hours using an overhead projector. We would then shuffle them in the carousel and make a second run. We would pick out distinguishing features of each fish—a spot here or a displaced fin there and then memorize the genus and species. Everyone in the group took turns until we all were comfortable with the identity of each jar. Needless to say, we all did well on the practical exam.

Unlike *ichthyology*, several of the zoology courses offered to pre-med students were clearly applicable to our later medical careers. One of these was histology. I signed up for histology in the last semester of my senior year. Professor Wilford had probably started teaching at the state university the same year as Professor Clare. At least my initial impression of him was that he was cut from the same mold. We of course used the manual he wrote for the *histology* laboratory. *Histology* (the study of human tissues) usually involves hours of having your retina fried by the intense light of a microscope. This is the preferred instrument of choice of the *pathologist* (the physician that studies tissues removed from live and deceased individuals). *Pathologists* are often relegated to the basement of hospitals where they peer through microscopes to diagnose whether an individual has cancer or what is causing a particular infection. Each student in our class was assigned a *slide set*—a series of glass slides neatly arranged in a large cardboard folder. Easy enough in our allotted lab time to go through these and identify all the right structures.

Of course, there always seemed to be that extra material that made completing the lab assignments in the scheduled time a Herculean effort. In this case, posters of *electron microscopy* (a very-high-resolution type of microscope) of various tissues were displayed around the room during each lab period. We were responsible for learning these at each lab session WHILE we were to review our glass slides. Solution: the Kodak idea worked so well with fish identification a few years earlier; why not a repeat performance? So the pre-med study group (which had now become quite the brotherhood for academic survival), decided to take turns at each lab session and photograph the posters. The weekend before the final practical, we all piled into our cars and headed to my parent's summer camp on the Gulf Coast. There we played the prescribed Russian roulette of slides in the Kodachrome carousel having never seen most of the posters during the lab sessions. Needless to say, our "learning aid" worked flawlessly at the time of the final practical.

In the fall of my senior year in college, it was time for the next step in my educational adventure. I had managed to maintain a respectful *GPA (grade point average)*. Most graduate-level education however requires at least three levels of assessment before one is admitted to a professional school—a review of the all-important *GPA* from college courses, a standardized entrance examination and a personal interview. The *Medical College Admissions Test* (*MCAT*) is the exam for entering medical school. As I think back, I am not sure why knowing a wide range of vocabulary or being able to solve complicated mathematical problems reflects my potential to evolve into a good physician. Perhaps being able to speak the king's English and being able to calculate proportions for drug dosage are useful. In any event, a good score on the *MCAT* exam is a pre-requisite for entrance into medical school. In fact, today, medical schools are often ranked nationally on the mean *GPA* and *MCAT* scores of their admission class of students. In any event, I took the peer-recommended Kaplan review course. It provided us with old test questions, vocabulary flash cards, and summary lectures given by graduate students. I don't remember my score on the *MCAT*, but I was accepted to both state medical schools and I was *wait-listed* at the one private medical school in the state. I really did not want to go to the private school anyway. I would probably have needed large student loans to pay for the tuition. I chose the older more established state medical school. Working every summer and getting half of my tuition and room and board support from my parents, I eventually only had to take out a $10,000 state loan for medical school expenses.

The tuition costs of higher education in our country have significantly outpaced inflation. Students are drawn to the allure of undergraduate school national rankings, often seeking out an *ivy league* or *little ivy* school. They may feel that this will enhance their chance for gaining entry into a premier medical school. A similar rationale is accepted for improving one's chance for selection into a top-notch residency training program. In 2016, the average U.S. graduating medical student carried a debt of $190,000 for their education[2]. *The Liaison Committee on Medical Education (LCME)* is the governing body that accredits all medical schools in the USA. Thus, all schools—both state-sponsored and private—must meet the same standards. Unlike a degree from Harvard or Yale law school that may result in a better career choice, most physicians are not judged on where they went to undergraduate school or medical school, but where they did their final clinical training. Medical schools are ranked annually by U.S. News and World Reports. The GPA and MCAT scores of the incoming medical student class, acceptance ratio, faculty-to-student ratios, assessment by residency directors, and research funding are parameters used for the ranking. The main two categories are research and primary care. Harvard, Johns Hopkins, and Yale usually top the list. I went to a state medical school—it was unranked in last year's report. Yet, I felt I received stellar education with little debt. And I believe I have managed to have an impact on health care in general during the course of my career.

There are currently four options for defraying the costs of a medical school education. The most common is the federal student loan program. Interest rates run between 6% and 7.5%. Interest payments can be deferred in some cases until after residency training. In other situations, *forbearance* can be used to allow the interest payments to accumulate and be added to the principal after one completes their training. The second option is to join one of the military services. This usually entails one year of service for every year of support once you complete residency training. A third option is a public service commitment. Loan forgiveness can be negotiated after one works in an underserved patient population area for two years after residency. Finally, there is the National Institutes of Health loan forgiveness program where one can apply for partial forgiveness of student loans for outstanding academic physician investigators. This allows them to remain at medical schools thus preventing the lure of private practice salaries.

This degree of debt for higher education is unstainable for the future of the health system in our country. Medical students understand that some subspecialties (invasive cardiology and orthopedics for example) have a higher earning potential than their primary care counterparts—general internal medicine and family practice. And so they are drawn to large metropolitan centers to practice these sub-specialties so they can enjoy some of the financial benefits of their hard-earned education. Thus, we continue to have a scarcity of primary care physicians, especially in the rural underserved areas of our vast country. Some relief may be in sight. Recently, one medical school in New York has announced that donors have created a foundation that will defray the annual $55,000 tuition for all current and future medical students at that institution[3]. They hope to attract the best medical student applicants with this promise.

3

Faced with Death for the First Time—Gross Anatomy

It seemed just a few years ago (now four and a half decades ago) that I walked into my first day of class at medical school in early July. There sat 175 future doctors—most hailed from the same state where the medical school was located. During the introductions, I was surprised to see eighteen of my high school classmates in the class. Most had gone to different pre-med university programs than the one I attended, but all had circled back home to enter the freshman class of medical school. This was probably not coincidental but instead, related to the high school prep education we had all received courtesy of the Jesuits.

Our first class was anatomy. We donned our plastic aprons—new and crisp, wrapped securely around our waists by a cloth strip that tied at the back. I realized that in the first twenty-four years of my life, I had never faced death. Here before me lay fifty stainless steel coffins—each elevated on four legs so that the tops were waist-high.

At each end was a large handle with two small chains that encircled pulleys. I found my assigned coffin number and introduced myself to the three other medical students who were to be my *lab partners*. Little did I know how many countless hours we would spend together in the next six months.

Our instructor appeared at the head of the room and announced that one of us should depress the handle at either end of the table. Almost simultaneously, the lids of the stainless steel coffins opened and fifty lost souls appeared to rise from their metal tombs. The *cadavers* lay face-down with a ghoulishly tan hue. The air in the room was immediately perfused with the strong odor of preserving fluid—a mixture of propylene glycol, phenol, ethanol, and glycerin[4].

Two of our classmates turned from their tables and exited the large wooden swinging doors at the entrance to the anatomy lab. They were never to be seen again.

There was an eerie quiet as our instructor admonished us, "These individuals have been gracious enough to donate their bodies so that you can learn from them. They are to be respected as the human beings they are. During the course of this class, you will become desensitized to their presence. Honor them as you would your own deceased family member."

We were instructed to wash the back of our cadaver. We decided "Joe" would be a good namesake. Then we opened our lab manuals and proceeded to begin the dissection to learn the innermost secrets of the human body just as our physician forefathers had done since the time of Vesalius in the 1500s[5]. As we cut into the skin on the back, we encountered our first muscle—the *trapezius*. Well, that's at least what it appeared to be based on the anatomy atlas called *Grant's Atlas of Anatomy* (our medical school decided to use this text as opposed to the well-known *Gray's Anatomy* used at many medical schools—the name later used for the popular television show).

With only two instructors assigned to the entire class, we soon realized that we were on our own—four young minds (Rick, Jeff, Dickie, and myself) and the newest edition of *Grant's Atlas of Anatomy*. It would be a long semester!

The lab period soon ended and we headed to lunch. Our hands and aprons smelled of phenol, and an oily residue (the glycerin) now stained our lab manuals. The cafeteria was serving roast beef that day. It seemed to look at lot like the trapezius muscle. Rick spoke first, "I think I'll go with chicken for lunch."

Ours was a traditional state medical school. Anatomy class was to consist of two one-and-a-half-hour lectures every week on Tuesday and Thursday and then three hours in the cadaver lab three times a week. There were four of us assigned to each cadaver for dissection. Luckily, the human body was conceived with a duplication of almost every organ system. This worked out perfectly for the anatomy lab. One member of the team at each side of the table was assigned to dissect, while the second member at his/her elbow read instructions from the lab manual. We were lucky—we were at the state medical school where there were more resources and lower tuition. Our colleagues across the street at the only private medical school in the state had six students assigned to each cadaver. Four would be in the lab and two had to rotate to the library to look at the albums of photos of the dissection.

Nine hours each week in the cadaver lab was hardly enough to keep up. Just when we felt that we were getting close to being on schedule with the next body system to be studied, we had fallen behind. This made for long extra hours at night and on the weekends to stay on pace. And then there were the *practicals*—the special exams for the anatomy lab. We always looked around for groups who had the best dissection since it was likely that the instructors would use their cadavers for a test *station*. The day of the first practical exam arrived. We were all assigned to a station at the starting gate. There were colored pins placed strategically in various structures with a card nearby containing a question. The problem was that the anatomical views never looked like the ones on our cadaver! And then there was that pesky buzzer that went off every two minutes followed by the instruction, "Move to the next station." This did not leave much time to contort our bodies to figure out where the colored pin was positioned at a particular station! The whole operation reminded me of the playing musical chairs at a kid's birthday party, except no one took a chair away the entire time!

One day, our lab group decided to take a break from our late evening dissection in the anatomy lab. What better adventure than to explore the part of the medical school building that was off-limits—the basement. Rumor had it that most of the cadavers in anatomy lab were unclaimed deceased patients from the nearby state hospital. They would first be embalmed, then submerged in a concrete pit of preservative until they were later retrieved for use in the cadaver lab. Our mission that evening was to find the "pit." We passed down dark passageways and opened old wooden doors until we finally arrived at a cavernous room. In the center was a sunken concrete structure that resembled a swimming pool filled with murky brown fluid. Spanning the ends were walk boards that were strategically placed to allow someone to cross the perimeter of the pit.

The silence was interrupted by the keeper of the pit—Jessie. "You boys don't belong down here ya know," he scolded.

"We just wanted to see where our cadaver came from," we replied.

"Well you found it. So go on with you, I don't want to see any of you fall in," he replied.

The "pit" had been part of the fifty-year history of the medical school. It was rumored never to have been drained and cleaned of all the human skin debris that had accumulated through the years.

Jessie, now realizing that he had a live audience that he can chat with, began the tale of a time when he had fallen into the pit. "Not a pleasant thing being covered with all that brown muck", he said. "The damnest thing though. When I was crawling out, my helper Billy came into the room. I reached out to him to give me a hand climbing out—but he looked at me with crazy eyes and took off running. Never saw the fella again—go figure."

We decided it was a good time to make our exit and return to our anatomy lab.

As part of our anatomy training, we were required to work at the city morgue for a session assisting the city coroner with autopsies. Saturday morning rolled around for our anatomy lab group's scheduled visit. As we strolled into the old building, we were greeted by the coroner—a portly gentleman who had obviously enjoyed much of the great Southern cuisine for which our city was famous. Our city also held another important distinction—we competed with Detroit for the title of the murder capital of the United States. We were escorted to a locker area and given our plastic aprons, goggles and masks. As we rounded the corner to the autopsy suite, we were astonished to see six nude bodies lying outside the room on the cement floor.

"Looks like the knife and gun club was busy last night," the coroner said. "And check out that last one," he said pointing to a female corpse. "She was just brought in."

I looked at her and realized she was not much older than myself. She lay on the cold concrete floor completely nude. She was still warm to the touch.

"Ok boys, here's the drill," the coroner instructed. "We are going to let you work in teams of two to do these autopsies. If you find a stab wound or a bullet hole, let me see it. If you get to find a bullet, dissect down to it, but do not touch it with an instrument. I need to take it out so that we can preserve the markings for forensic analysis."

And so it went for the next four hours. Our team found four bullets that day. We left exhausted but decisive that pathology would not be our future calling as a medical subspecialty.

Towards the end of the semester, we were all given five- by eight-sized index cards that gave us a brief history of our cadaver's demise. Most of the notes were cryptic—an age and a brief diagnosis like *pneumonia* or *renal failure*. Our card describing Joe's untimely death was virtually blank—"forty-eight years of age; cause of death—unknown." Jeff looked at me and grinned. We of course did not perceive ourselves to be hot-shot forensic pathologists after our brief episode at the coroner's office. But, we did know what we had discovered when our group had approached the chest dissection of our cadaver. Rick was assigned to "run the saw." After all we wanted him to be proficient as he had declared orthopedics to be his future interest in medicine. He carefully used the small saw to cut open the ster*num* (breast bone) from the set of ribs on each side.

"What the heck," Rick exclaimed as he elevated the sternum from its anatomical location. To our amazement, a we saw a four-inch knife blade protruding through the bone into the chest cavity. We didn't need an index card to inform us how Bill died—it was obvious to even this group of first-year medical students.

When I was in the thick of anatomy class, I wondered why there was a prescribed sequence of the dissection of our cadaver. As I mentioned earlier, we started with the back muscles on the first day. Other parts did not follow in any logical order. The face came later—perhaps to allow us to be desensitized in our experience with our deceased "Joe"? Of course, a cadaver face is dehydrated from the formaldehyde and does not look anything like a normal person. The skin is leathery and the eyes are cloudy. Once we were finished with the facial muscles and nerves, it was on to the brain. To study the brain, one must first open the bony *calvarium* (skull) that protects it from outside insults.

"Let me have the saw," Rick said. "After all, I am the future bone doctor in our group."

With that Rick proceeded to use the bone saw to make a circular cut around the *calvarium*. After removing the top of the skull, we all gazed in at how nicely "Joe's" brain was nestled in its protective cocoon. Weeks later, it was time to dissect the hand. The hand was relegated to the last phase of the dissection. I could not help but feel empathy for the human who lay before us who was once alive when I grasped our "Joe's" hand with my own. And yet the hand is one of the most marvelous of God's many creations. There are twenty-nine different joints in the hand. Intricate pulleys and tendons allow the last four digits to be flexed and extended by muscles that are located a distance away in the forearm. Muscles intrinsic to the hand itself allow the thumb to *oppose* or move across the palm. This *opposable thumb* makes us unique in the animal world and has allowed *homo sapiens* to evolve and learn to use tools. As one dissects the marvels of the hand, one realizes why today's engineers are having such difficulties in creating a robotic equivalent. Dissecting the hand last helped me embrace the humanity of 'Joe" that we had come to know during the previous four months. We would miss him. He was our first of many patients who would unselfishly offer themselves in our learning process to become a physician.

Throughout the challenges of higher education, study groups of diverse individuals coalesce to more effectively conquer the stress and challenges of academia. Our band of brothers was dubbed the "banana bunch." We were given this label after a prank that occurred during a boring lecture class on clinical diagnosis. At lunch one day, Rick decided to purchase a cluster of six bananas from the little lady that sold fruit from her truck that she always parked in front of the city hospital. As we sat in the back row of the lecture hall (the usual residence for our study group), he realized that the slide projector was just above our heads. Although not a pre-planned stunt, Rick fixed the bananas to a mop handle. At the opportune moment when our instructor had his back to the screen in the front of the lecture hall, Rick elevated the fruity cluster in front of the projector. Much to the amusement of our medical student class, a silhouette of the bunch of bananas appeared on the lecture screen. For the next several weeks, a staff with the cluster of bananas atop marked the reserved seating on the back row for the "banana bunch."

The members of the "banana bunch" were diverse in our future aspirations in medicine. I wanted to go into OB-GYN, while Ken and Jeff thought anesthesiology was their calling. Rick aspired to orthopedic surgery and Dickie (the most intellectual of the group) wanted to be an ophthalmologist. The general consensus was that the "bottom" of the medical school class ranking went into obstetrics or orthopedics—Rick and I didn't care. Ken (an aspiring anesthesiologist) was one of the most unique members of our group. We were all envious as he had a "photographic memory." While the rest of the banana bunch labored for weeks over texts and notes for the written exams in anatomy, Ken made it his mission to acquire as many of the old medical school tests that he could find. The night before the big exam, he would stay up and memorize all the questions and the correct answers.

"The human body has not evolved that much over the past few years," he would instruct us. "How many different ways can you ask questions on the same human anatomy anyway?"

He of course was correct. While the rest of us peered out the windows during the exam to see if some divine inspiration could help us with the answers, Ken smirked as he recognized each of the questions. Of course, he was always the first to turn in his exam. I thought this was the easy way out. How could he be confident as a physician if he did not really know human anatomy. The truth was he would eventually only really need to know where to place a breathing tube into the patient's windpipe to put them to sleep for surgery.

As I would come to learn in my career, many of the things we memorized in medical school would not prove useful in my later years as a practicing physician. I still remember the useless fact that there are twenty-one amino acids that make up all the proteins in the human body. This knowledge has never turned out to be crucial to my caring for patients.

The curriculum at our medical school was a traditional format—the first two years were didactic lectures and the third and fourth years were clinical rotations at hospitals. The only clinical exposure was in the second year when we were assigned to go to the hospital to perform practice history and physicals. At the end of clinical diagnosis class, we would have to take a practical examination where we were assigned a group of select patients picked by the instructor. Rumor had it that he recruited certain patients over the years with abnormal findings. We were all on our toes. One patient was supposed to have glass eye. If you noted the usual *pupils equal and reactive to light*—you failed. Another patient was supposed to have his heart located on the right side of his chest (called *dextrocardia*) as compared to the usual location on the left side. No one in our group was stumped by the trick patients.

We still longed for exposure to patients. Wasn't that why we decided to go to medical school? Then Ken in the banana bunch (the same guy who seemed to have all the connections to secure old anatomy tests) found out that second-year medical students could go to the emergency room on one particular night and the surgery residents would allow them to suture lacerations. Our city has an annual Mardi Gras celebration—it is a tradition consisting of a major day of revelry just before the forty days of sacrifice that begins during the Catholic Lent season. Many patrons of the event partake of a little too much alcohol and miss a step on the street curb. A fall and a head laceration are often the result. Based on Ken's reconnaissance, four of us donned our lab coats and headed to the emergency room at the city hospital at around 8 p.m. Mardi Gras night. We soon found one of the surgery interns who was suturing a head laceration on an inebriated forty-five-year-old man.

"Can I help you guys?" he asked.

"We heard we can come help suture tonight," Ken responded. "Do you have any cases we can do?"

The intern pointed to two rows of chairs holding more than twenty patients. Most were slumped over with dried blood on their faces.

"That's the waiting line," he responded. "Have any of you sutured before?"

"No, but we are quick learners," I responded.

"Ok, watch me do this one," he responded.

We all peered over his shoulder as he irrigated the patient's head wound with peroxide, then injected the edges of a four-inch laceration with a local anesthetic. He then expertly placed several nylon interrupted sutures, tying them by circling the needle holder first clockwise then counter-clockwise around the end of the suture.

"No need for a dressing or antibiotics. The scalp has a great blood supply and rarely do these get infected," the intern instructed. "Tell them to keep it dry for two days and come back to clinic in five days to have the sutures removed. Oh, and if you see bone or if the laceration is deep enough to go through a tough white connective tissue layer, come get me. Otherwise, have at it."

We all looked at each other in amazement. Whatever happened to the old medical adage, "See one, do one, teach one"? We had skipped the middle step. We each set about organizing a suture station and went to work. In two hours, it was standing room only in the suture waiting room. I think I sutured more than twenty lacerations that night. Toward the end of my experience, I even started trimming the edges of the more jagged cuts with a scalpel to make a clean line for healing with minimal scar. We all left exhausted a 6 a.m. This was truly our first night *on call*. We were real doctors now!

4

So You Want To Be
An Obstetrician?

Our state school followed the traditional model of medical education at the time. The first two years were pre-clinical classes—lots of
memorization in anatomy, biochemistry, histology, pharmacology,
pathology, and more. There was an introduction to clinical medicine
course where we were sent to the hospital to practice the basics of
history and physical examination. This was followed in the third year
by four twelve-week rotations in the hospital—medicine, surgery,
pediatrics, and obstetrics/gynecology. Senior year was for electives,
although a rotation on psychiatry was required. Summers were free
and most of us spent them working to help pay for tuition and room
and board (I spent summers working in the offshore kitchens of a
major oil company).

Today's medical school curriculum has evolved over time.
Courses in the first two years are mixed with clinical correlation
lectures—the part of the anatomy lab associated with the female

reproductive organs might include lectures from a practicing obstetrician/gynecologist. Required rotations are much shorter (four – six weeks) and the student must pass a *shelf* exam, a national standardized written test, in each specialty. The exam score is used with the assessment of the clinical mentors to derive a final grade for a rotation. There is time for elective rotations even in the third year. There are some advantages to this approach as many students are not sure where they are headed later in their medical training and want to "test drive" a subspecialty before deciding on residency training (where you actually learn the practice of medicine). Students take a national board exam in the basic sciences (*USMLE* step one) at the end of their second year of medical school. They must pass the *USMLE* step two exam by the end of their fourth year in order to graduate. This involves one day of written questions on clinical medicine followed by a one-day practical on patient assessment. Most medical students do not take summers off and complete their clinical rotations midway through their fourth year. They then use the last six months to study for boards.

The newest medical schools are implementing an even more novel model of education. Traditional memorization courses are being replaced by interactive problem-solving sessions that include a team approach with nursing and pharmacy students. The rationale is that medical information today is readily available through computer searches even on smartphones. A public service project modeled on a new innovative idea designed by the student is required in the later medical school years. In fact, a recent survey of U.S. medical students found that 24% admitted to almost never attending formal lectures at their school and instead chose to view these recorded lectures online[6]. More time was spent instead "studying for boards." Only time will tell if these changes will produce a better educated and compassionate physician workforce. Unfortunately, many of these modifications have been implemented with little subsequent study as to whether they are achieving the desired goal.

My third year of medical school began in July with the start of one of four required clinical rotations. I chose to start with obstetrics and gynecology since this was the specialty I was considering for my future career. I sometimes wonder what peaked my interest in obstetrics. After all, I had no previous life experiences with pregnancy or childbirth. There was no OB-GYN physician in my family. Perhaps it was the influence of two of my best friends in college—Amy and Kathy. Amy had dated one of my high school classmates and had ended up at the same state university where I went to undergraduate school. I met Kathy through Amy. The three of us spent many long hours over chocolate chip malts pondering where life would take us.

"You are so easy to talk to," said Amy one day. "You should consider being an OB-GYN. You would be good at it."

I decided to do my OB-GYN clinical rotation in another city than where our medical school was located, so I ended up at the inner-city hospital in the capital of our state. The rumor was that the medical students were given more responsibilities there. On the first day, all of the OB-GYN medical students were shown a film on how to deliver a baby. Now, this was a brand-new experience for me since I had never even seen a delivery before. I then packed up my belongings and head out for the twelve-week rotation.

The next day I arrived at the hospital named after one of our former governors. Our group of medical students was assigned to go to the medical education office for our ID badges and white coats In general, the tradition in medicine at that time was that the length of the white coat was directly related to the years of training. The medical student wore a waist-high coat, while the resident wore a coat to the mid-thigh and the attending physician's coat ended below the knees. Unlike the length of the coat, the number of accessories placed in the pockets of the coat is inversely related to the accumulated number of years of training. The medical student typically carries a stethoscope, an *oto-ophthalmoscope* (a device used to look into a patient's eyes and ears), and several paperback reference manuals. The attending, on the other hand, will often have to ask the medical student to use their stethoscope because his/her pockets are empty.

Much to our surprise, we received mid-thigh length coats on our new obstetrical rotation—just like the residents. We were also supplied with pagers or *beepers* so that the nurses could find us at all times. We felt like real doctors now!

I was overwhelmed with excitement when it came time for me to deliver my very first baby. The OB resident stood next to me to provide coaching on the various maneuvers I would need to undertake.

"Let the head deliver, allow it to *restitute* (turn naturally so that the back of the head was on the same side as the baby's shoulders), put your hands above and below the head, then pull down, pull up, then flip the baby onto your arms so you can cut the umbilical cord."

Seemed easy enough. Babies have come into this world since the first cavewoman delivered a child with far less instruction! With a primeval scream, my patient pushed her first baby out, barely giving me enough time to catch his slippery little body as he was headed toward the *kick bucket* on the floor. The *kick bucket* is the name given to the metal container at the foot of the delivery bed used to collect the blood and amniotic fluid that results from a vaginal delivery. Since it was located near the obstetrician's feet, it became dubbed the *kick bucket*. Today it has been replaced by special drapes that have a bag to collect these fluids.

"An *F* for effort on that delivery," the resident said.

Was this what I really wanted to do for the rest of my life? I left that day totally dejected. Maybe like Rick, a member of the banana bunch, orthopedics would be my ultimate calling. After all I had become pretty skilled with a hammer in my summer jobs as a carpenter.

I returned to the hospital the next day with a newfound enthusiasm. My second delivery that day went much better—it was "controlled" as they say. I still could not quite figure out that "flip the baby on your arm thing" maneuver. This would also be my first night of in-house call on the obstetrical service. The unique thing about our medical student experience on the OB service was that we did all the deliveries at night by ourselves under the direction of the senior night nurses. Residents were only to be awakened for C-sections. Consistent with clinical practice at the time, most women underwent a procedure known as *episiotomy*—a surgical incision performed on the outer vagina just as the head was about to deliver to prevent catastrophic tearing of the pregnant woman's tissues. There are two basic types of episiotomies—*midline* and *mediolateral*. The midline *episiotomy* is made right in the middle but if it extends then the *rectal sphincter* (the muscle that encircles the rectum) can be lacerated. This requires a fairly sophisticated repair to maintain *anal continence* (the ability to control the loss of feces and flatus). The *mediolateral episiotomy* is cut on a forty-five-degree angle (interesting that one can tell if the delivering physician is right or left-handed based on which side of the patient the incision is made). It almost never extends into the *rectal sphincter* but can extend deep into the patient's buttocks. Once thought to be a prophylactic procedure to prevent excessive stretching of female tissues at the time of a vaginal delivery, the *episiotomy* has fallen into disfavor in modern obstetrical practice. More recent studies have shown that its original purpose was unproven and spontaneous *lacerations* (tears) of the birth canal have fewer consequences for the pregnant patient. At our hospital, medical students were not allowed to perform *midline episiotomies* since this might entail waking the sleeping resident if there was an extension to perform the more complicated repair. With no previous instruction, I performed my first *mediolateral episiotomy* that first night on call. As per the nurse's direction, I had injected a local anesthetic into the area. Using the "typical" sutures that were handed to me, I began to repair what turned out to be a complex laceration. When a surgeon cuts across tissue planes on a forty-five-degree angle, the body has a tendency to retract these tissues. This makes lining up the tissues into their original anatomical location quite difficult. After about forty-five minutes of work, I had completed my first repair.

The nurse looked over my work and commented "not what it used to look like. Try again."

So, I took out all the sutures, reinjected the area with local anesthetic, and proceeded with a second attempt. An hour later, I had now achieved a "much better" approval from my nurse. Later I taught myself that I could place one suture at the edge of the skin between the vagina and the outer skin and just hold this to line up all the other tissues. Then while holding this suture as a handle, I could approximate all of the other tissues much better. Plastic surgery at its best!

Befriending the night nurses was a must for learning. The labor ward was an open room with six beds separated only by curtains. I soon realized that I should first "check" the patient to assess the *degree of dilation* of the cervix (the assessment of how labor was progressing). Then I would ask the night nurse to check them again to see how accurate my assessment had been. Before long I was quite skilled at determining the *degree of cervical dilation*.

Once it was determined that the patient was in labor (you usually had to be at least four centimeters dilated to be a "keeper"), the patient was admitted to the labor ward. Next, a little old lady appeared behind the curtains to administer the prep and enema. All patients were shaved from their breasts to their knees for "cleanliness" I was instructed. They then received a "triple H enema—high, hot, and hella-of-a-lot." This consisted of a one-liter bag of warm normal saline placed very high up on the IV pole to allow it to run in. The rationale was that it can't be a good thing to have a newborn exposed to its mom's feces as it comes out of the birth canal.

One night, I heard our attendant who did all the preps screaming at one of the new laboring patients, "You hold it, dammit. Hold it."

After a few minutes, I peered behind the drape to see the frustrated prep lady holding the enema tubing in her hand with a bed full of water between the patient's legs.

"Can I have a look?" I asked. Now this particular patient was of a generous habitus. I followed the enema tube and noted that it had not been inserted into the rectum but into the patient's vagina instead.

I placed it into the proper orifice and turned to the prep lady— "let's give it another try."

The OB-GYN clinical service was quite busy. Days were spent in the operating room assisting with gynecologic procedures—hysterectomies, tubal ligations, and other operations. And then there were OB and GYN outpatient clinics. Night call was every third night on Labor and Delivery Unit for the three-month rotation. This meant going without sleep the following day until our work was completed the next afternoon. We never talked about being *post-call*—a common term used by today's residents. We simply slept very well the evening we finally got home. But these long hours in the hospital allowed us to gain incredible experience. By the end of my OB rotation, I had delivered fifty-six babies. This is a marked contrast to today's medical student who on questioning at interviews for an obstetrical residency position will brag that they had delivered four *placentas* (the afterbirth) during their core obstetrical rotation. I sometimes wonder how they decided that this was the right specialty for them for the rest of their medical career!

On one of my last nights on call, I was checking a patient who was reported to be close to *term* (the end of her pregnancy). She was four centimeters dilated, but the fetal head felt awfully small on my vaginal exam. Ultrasound (today a routine part of obstetrical practice with equipment on every Labor and Delivery Unit) was still an undiscovered technology that had not yet been introduced into the field of obstetrics.

I asked my senior night nurse "Do you think she could have twins?"

"Good thought," she replied.

"Then what should we do?" I asked.

"An X ray will tell for sure," she said. I quickly placed my patient in a wheelchair and whisked her to radiology.

"Need a stat film of the abdomen," I said. A few minutes later, the tech brought out the developed film from the darkroom. Twins— the first head down and the second *breech* (feet first). Elated, I rushed the patient back to Labor and Delivery.

A minute later, I threw open the door to the resident call room. "Twins," I announced "and in advanced labor."

The OB resident jumped out of bed and ran with me to the labor ward. The nurses had already moved the patient to the delivery room. Moments later the head of the first twin was *crowning*.

"You deliver this one," the resident said. "Your reward for a good diagnosis."

After the first twin was born, the resident reached in and grabbed the second twin by his feet. Just a few seconds later, two newborn brothers had entered the world. Elated at the outcome, I knew obstetrics was my calling!

During elective clinical rotations in the last year of medical school, many students seek a rotation at another medical school where they are interested in applying for a residency training position. These rotations are known as *AIs (acting internships)* because the student is allowed to have more advanced clinical responsibilities based on their previous training in medical school. This gives the student a competitive edge over other applicants who are not well known to the program. After doing some research, I decided to do one of these month-long AI rotations at another premier southern medical school. I rented an apartment (which I rarely saw except to sleep) and dedicated myself to work hard to impress the attending physicians. After all, this was known to be a great residency program for training in OB-GYN.

Dr. Charlie Rose was the Chairman—a well-known figure in academic circles in the field of obstetrics. His academic office was an intimidating sight. You were surrounded by the head mounts of large game animals that he had hunted from around the world. The rumor was that in lieu of a financial honorarium for invited lectures, Charlie would prefer to be paid with a hunting or fishing trip.

I worked hard on the rotation volunteering for night call every third night. I had a clear advantage over the local medical students. Their obstetrical required rotation was not scheduled until their fourth year so they were naïve to obstetrics. I had already done my fair share of deliveries. I did another thirty-five deliveries and was even instructed by the local OB-GYN residents on how to perform *outlet forceps* (the placement of special instruments to help pull a baby

43

from the birth canal when the mother is having difficulty pushing it out on her own).

On one occasion, I was in the midst of performing a delivery, when Dr. Rose, the Chairman, walked in. "Son, I want to see you get on your knees to visualize that posterior shoulder coming out if you are going to do this delivery right."

Without hesitation, I genuflected to complete the delivery. I later learned that he did not realize I was an *AI* but thought I was a family practice resident on an obstetrical rotation. When he was made aware of this fact, I was summoned to his office.

"Son, you are aware of the rules of the match that forbid me from promising you a position," he said. "That being said, our program only takes six residents in OB-GYN. We would be VERY interested in you applying here." I was interested too.

Obstetrical forceps have an interesting history[7]. First designed by the Chamberlain family in England in the late 1600s, the brothers managed to keep their trade secret by only transporting the instruments in a gilded box. When they were called to employ the forceps for a difficult delivery, the pregnant woman was blind-folded and the instruments applied under the cover of a blanket. The Chamberlain's forceps were not divulged for almost a century until one of their descendants was rumored to sell a set to a Dutch obstetrician. Although over 600 different variations were ultimately developed (most are named for the physician who invented them), today there are only fifteen to twenty different types remaining in clinical use. The basic instrument consists of two metal blades that encircle the fetal head. After the placement of each individual blade into the vagina, the blades are engaged by a locking mechanism just above the handles. Traction is applied by the obstetrician while the patient pushes. Forceps are classified as *outlet, low or mid*, based on how far down the birth canal the fetal head has descended into the mother's pelvis. They are typically used when the *second stage of labor* (the period between complete cervical dilation to ten centimeters and delivery of the fetus) becomes prolonged or the pregnant woman becomes exhausted during voluntary pushing with contractions. Today, the lack of instruction by senior obstetricians on the correct forceps technique has resulted in a virtual abandonment of *mid-forceps* deliveries in lieu of Cesarean section. In addition, *outlet forceps* are being routinely replaced by *vacuum extraction*. In this technique, a small plastic cup is attached to the rear of the presenting fetal head and after a vacuum is created with a hand pump, traction is applied to the handle. Data has indicated that forceps deliveries are more often associated with maternal injury to the vagina, while vacuum deliveries are more often associated with fetal injury (typically bleeding under the scalp).

The time had come in the fall of my final year of medical school to arrange interviews for residency—the next four years of my training. I looked through the catalogs of the various OB-GYN residencies to see where I could get the best training. If only there had been a Google search, but of course the internet was not even a concept yet! I had always lived in the deep south so all of the programs I selected were located below the *Mason-Dixon* line (that boundary that separated the Southern states from the Northern states in the Civil War). The residency program affiliated with my state medical school was one of my considerations. A plus was its association with large training hospitals that cared primarily for indigent patients. A negative was that the residents had to rotate to four different cities in the state over the course of the four-year training program. I carefully planned out a two-week trip to cover all the programs that peaked my interest.

I would start with a brief visit with the Chairman of OB-GYN at our own school—Dr. Abe. On the scheduled day of my personal interview, I dressed in my best suit and arrived at the chair's office early. After waiting for almost an hour, his secretary came out to inform me that the Chairman had left town unexpectedly and I would have to reschedule. As I was leaving, I glanced back to see Dr. Abe walking out of his office. Disheartened, I decided it was probably better to go elsewhere for my residency anyway to get a better perspective of health care outside of my native state. It would later tun out to be one of the best decisions I ever made in my medical career.

My parents were middle class, and as I was one the oldest of five boys, I learned not to spend money frivolously. I purchased a *tour America* pass from Greyhound that let me grab a bus to any city in continental USA. Some of my interviews were only a day apart. In these cases, I would schedule a plane flight between cities. I stayed in *Days Inn* hotels over the course of the two weeks and washed my underwear and socks in the sink. As I neared the end of my interviews, I arrived at my final destination. My bags had been lost by the airlines. I would not have a suit for the interview. All I had was the polo shirt, jeans, and tennis shoes that I was wearing. Should I cancel my interview? It was early Sunday and my interview was scheduled the following morning. And then an epiphany—I would rent a tux! So off I went in a cab to the local men's formal wear rental.

"A powder blue tux with a ruffled shirt is our most popular rental," the salesperson said.

"For proms or residency interviews?" I asked. The next morning, I showed up in my blue tux and patent leather shoes. Of course, I had to tell my story of lost baggage many times that morning. But it was clear that I was scoring points with my interviewers regarding my ability to problem solve on short notice. At least I would stand out when the selection committee met to choose their final six candidates for the residency.

I especially liked this OB-GYN residency program. The trainee would get a chance to work at the university medical center, a large private hospital, and an inner-city hospital—all in the same city! I was conflicted. My previous *AI* rotation at the southern medical school allowed me to determine that it too would be great choice for residency training. I had impressed them with my work ethic and my clinical skills. I would be a *shoe in* to be selected there. But I really liked this last program. How was I to decide?

Two weeks later I decided to return to the location of my last interview. I arrived unannounced on a Friday afternoon with a small overnight bag and declared, "I am a visiting medical student interested in the residency program. I want to see what the program is really like in the eyes of the residents."

I would first take call at the university hospital. Jean, a second year OB-GYN resident, welcomed me. She was an impressive resident with an air of confidence about her. I tagged along like a new puppy. As the midnight hour approached, we were called *stat* by the nurses in Labor and Delivery. When we entered the room, we were greeted by a wide-eyed intern who had just completed the vaginal delivery of a patient having her fourth baby. The floor at the foot of the patient's delivery bed was covered in blood. A strange mass, clearly foreign to me, protruded from between the patient's legs.

"I really did not pull that hard," stated the intern.

"Uterine prolapse," said Jean and she kicked into high gear. Before I could blink, she donned a gown and gloves and then she calmly placed the uterus back inside the patient into its normal anatomical position.

With her hand remaining in place, she ordered, "Methergine IM now and run that pit wide open." And as quickly as the events had transpired, all had been resolved, and a calm returned to the room. Jean removed her hand and the uterine bleeding stopped. I was impressed.

After my adrenaline high wore off, I decided to head to the call room to grab some sleep. The next morning, I showered, grabbed some breakfast in the hospital cafeteria, and hailed a cab. I was headed to the inner-city hospital for another night on call.

I was greeted by John Lang, the second-year resident who could only be described as a clone of the *fat man* from the book *The House of God*. John was worldly, confident, and the nurses revered him. He was in charge of the entire hospital for any OB-GYN problem. It was Saturday and unusually quiet. The five-bed ward for Labor and Delivery had only three patients in labor. All patients labored in one room and were then transferred to the delivery room for the actual delivery of the baby.

As the evening progressed, we followed the labor of one particularly large woman. She had delivered two other children but John performed *Leopold's maneuvers* (a placing of the hands on the patient's pregnant belly to guess at the baby's weight).

"This one will be a keeper. Surely bigger than your last two," he told the panting patient. An hour later she was *complete* and the nurses wheeled her into the delivery room. She reluctantly moved over to the delivery bed between contractions and placed her legs in stirrups.

With the next uterine contraction, she screamed, "It's coming!". The baby's head popped out before John had even a chance to turn around from putting on his gloves. It seemed to retract back against the patient's body—almost like a turtle's head returning to its shell when it realizes there is danger lurking.

"Shoulder dystocia," John declared. "Crank those legs back" he ordered to the nurses who promptly removed the patient's two legs from the stirrups and bent them towards the patient's head. A tug on the head and it did not budge. This was all new to me even though I had done almost ninety deliveries in my short career. John expertly reached inside the vagina below the baby's head and found the baby's *posterior* arm (the arm closest to the patient's back). In one swift movement he brought it out. The shoulders slid out and he was then able to pull on the head and deliver this ten-pound two ounce bouncing baby boy with ease. Wow, I was impressed. And not even a bead of sweat on John's forehead! These residents at this program knew what they are doing. And the pathology!

I retired exhausted to the call room later that evening. The next morning, I headed to the airport to return home. On the flight back I decided I was no longer conflicted—I wanted to come to this program. I would match them number one. I only hoped they remembered the medical student with the blue tuxedo!

The final step in my medical school training was to take the *Federal Licensing Exam (FLEX)*. This was the predecessor to the current *United States Medical Licensing Exam (USLME)*. This would be the first of the eleven standardized tests I would ultimately be required to pass during the course of my medical career. The test was given over two days and involved questions about various clinical patients with diverse medical problems. After passing, I received a license in the mail from my state—technically I could *hang out a shingle* and practice medicine as a general physician.

One of the major stressful times for all medical students occurs in the spring of their final year—the *match*. Most folks know about the NBA, NFL, and fantasy football drafts. A not-too-dissimilar process matches medical students to residency training positions (also called *graduate medical education or graduate medical education [GME]* positions). Medical students interview at various residency training programs for a three- to four-year training position where they truly learn their profession. The *match* is performed by a computerized algorithm. The institution tries to *rank* the top applicants to get the best trainees, while the medical student *ranks* his/her top training positions. In early March of each year, the residents receive their assignments. There are several rules. The institutions cannot make any promises to guarantee a position outside of the *match* and the medical student must accept the decision of the match.

Match day is a big celebration at most medical schools. Parents and friends attend the ceremony and the envelopes are placed on a bulletin board. Once the envelope is opened, there are shouts of glee from spouses (this is where they will be living for the next four years of their life) and tears of disappointment when a student does not get his/her first or second *choice*. Most medical students get their first top one to three choices for a training position. Unfortunately, there are more medical students that graduate from U.S. medical schools than there are *GME* positions in residency training. The day before the *match* results are announced, medical students that do not match to a residency position are notified of the remaining unmatched open positions across the country. They then *scramble* to see if they can secure a position at one of these institutions.

Most of the *GME* positions for residents are supported by the federal government as part of Part B of Medicare payments to hospitals. Some states add additional funding for primary care GME residency positions. One may question why federal tax revenue is used to educate physicians. The average medical *intern* (the first year of residency training) today makes $12.70/hour in salary, not that much above the current national minimum wage of $7.25/hour. Of course, this is much improved as compared to the calculated $8.70/hour I was paid as a resident. Since residency training occurs at many hospitals that care for an underserved patient population, federal funds in essence support these residents for providing medical care while they are perfecting their clinical skills.

Truth be known, I don't remember my match day. I think my school put the envelop in my mailbox. I did match to my first choice for residency. The blue tux had paid off!

5

Starting Out—The Intern Year

The term *intern* was coined from the French word *interne* which meant assistant doctor. The establishment of formal clinical training in medicine occurred at Johns Hopkins in 1889. One of the three founding teaching physicians, William Halstead, is credited with the initial use of the word intern to describe first year trainees in 1904[8]. In 1975, *the U.S. Accreditation Council for Graduate Medical Education* decided to drop the term and call first-year trainees *residents*[9]. The term *resident* (sometimes also referred to as *house officer*) has a more interesting history in American medicine. Early trainees were offered housing in the hospital with meals provided in the hospital cafeteria. As such these trainees *resided* in the hospital. Many training programs prohibited marriage. Stipends were meager—about $300/month (calculated to be five cents/hour taking into account the total number of hours worked each week).

When I started by first year of post medical school training, we were still called *interns*. I guess it's difficult to relinquish a term that has been in use for almost a century. Today resident applicants match to a four-year OB-GYN residency program, although for those who have difficulty matching, there are positions known as *transitional internships* that are only one year in length. During that year, these trainees rotate through many different clinical services. In essence, even though I had matched to an obstetrics and gynecology residency, my schedule resembled a transitional internship: only four months of obstetrics and then clinical rotations in internal medicine, neonatal intensive care, ward surgery, and emergency room surgery. My intern class consisted of five men and one woman. This is a far cry from today's OB-GYN intern class where 85% of OB-GYN interns are women[10]. The reason for this dramatic shift is perplexing. In 2019, for the first time women outnumbered men in the entering class of U.S. medical schools[11]. Perhaps it is the association of women with pregnancy itself that leads them to choose OB-GYN (pediatrics is the second highest specialty with a predominance of women in current clinical practice, 58% in 2020)[12]. Or perhaps it is the notion that continues to permeate the OB-GYN specialty that women only want to see female physicians. This has led male medical students to choose other surgical specialties like orthopedics or urology with better career opportunities once they complete their medical school training. In truth, my experience over the past forty years has indicated that women want a compassionate physician that they can trust. The gender of the physician does not matter.

My first clinical rotation in my intern year was obstetrics. My fellow intern, also named Ken, and I were on every other night call for two months—thirty hours in the hospital and eighteen hours off. A true biphasic life cycle. There are 168 hours in a seven-day week; we worked on average one hundred nine hours or 65% of the week.

I had been on service for about six weeks when I awoke one day to realize I was fully clothed in my bed. I looked at my bedside clock and the digital display read 5:50. My clock did not have an AM or PM indicator (this technical attribute would be introduced to society at a later date).

I thought to myself, "Oh, God I feel asleep and I'm late for morning rounds" (I usually started morning rounds in the hospital at 6 a.m.). Or maybe I had just fallen asleep after call and it was close to 6 p.m. *Which was it? I thought in a panic.*

I hurried outside to see if it was dawn or dusk. No good—I could not figure which direction was west and which was east to use the sun as an indicator.

I turned on my T.V. "And that's the evening news for another day. This is Walter Cronkite signing off," I heard the television anchor state. I was safe. A snack and then back to bed after setting the alarm for the next morning.

Residents today have the benefit of many ancillary support services—patient transport, intravenous line placement services, *phlebotomy* technicians (drawing blood samples), and lab testing. These are commodities that did not exist in my residency. Many times, especially at the inner-city hospital, we were required to wheelchair our patients to the X-ray department. We became very adept at drawing blood samples and starting intravenous lines. Even at the university hospital, when we admitted a pregnant patient with premature labor, we routinely performed bacterial cultures of the cervix for certain bacteria. We then had to take the swabs to a small satellite laboratory and plate them on *blood agar* (the plastic dishes that allowed the bacteria to grow). The gonorrhea culture plate was placed in a jar, a candle lit, and placed in the jar and then the top screwed on. This depleted the oxygen in the bottle as the candle burned out so that this bug could grow better. All the cultures were then put in a small warm incubator in the lab to be picked up by the *microbiology* lab the next morning. Probably the most common test we performed was to look for *ferning*. When a pregnant patient thinks her bag of waters (*amniotic fluid*) is leaking, she is at risk for infection and a decision has to be made about delivery. Amniotic fluid forms a beautiful snow-flake-like pattern when it dries on a glass slide. These patients had a speculum placed in their vagina and a swab was taken. The swab was then rolled over a glass slide and we looked under the microscope for *ferning*. A piece of *nitrazine pH* paper (used to detect the level of acid) was rubbed across the back of the speculum once it was removed. A blue color meant that the acid level was low—another confirmation that amniotic fluid was present. Residents today no longer are allowed to perform these tests.

The *Clinical Laboratory Improvement Act (CLIA)* was passed into law in 1988[13]. The intent was to regulate the quality of results from commercial and diagnostic laboratories. Unfortunately, *CLIA* regulations found their way to bedside testing also known as *point-of-care testing*—those diagnostic tests that were quickly performed by clinicians to make rapid decisions about patient care. Today, nitrazine paper and the microscope have been removed from OB unit because it is almost impossible to meet the CLIA regulations for assessing quality control with so many individuals performing the tests. An expensive monoclonal antibody test is used to check for leaking amniotic fluid. It costs almost $500 per test—a far cry from the cost of a glass slide and a piece of pH paper!

I had done my fair share of routine vaginal deliveries as a medical student. I had assisted in several C-sections during my clinical rotations, but I had never held the *scalpel*—that metal knife handle with a disposable sharp surgical blade. After about a week on Labor and Delivery, the chief OB resident felt it was time to let me do my first C-section. I remember being a chief resident and later an attending physician. Supervising a novice surgeon that rarely knows how to even correctly hold the scalpel can be a trying experience. It requires patience and fortitude. July was always the month in obstetrics when I would perspire the most at the operating room table during these teaching cases. Unfortunately, there is no other way for the intern to learn how to do an operation. There is no simulation lab or a pig lab for practice C-section procedures. You just have to jump in and swim. For the patient's sake, there is always a lifeguard on duty to rescue you—the more experienced surgeon across the table. Dr. Dan Folger was my chief resident. A few weeks earlier he had been a third-year-level OB-GYN resident, so Dan was still learning how to be a chief resident in this early part of July. My patient was a twenty-four-year-old woman who was having her second baby. This one was much larger than the last and she had experienced an arrest of the dilation of her cervix at six centimeters. The head was just too big to fit through her pelvic bones. Her diagnosis was *cephalopelvic disproportion*. We would have to deliver the baby by C-section. The spinal anesthetic was already in place. The operating room nurses had cleansed the skin with a brown antiseptic solution called *betadine*. They had placed a small tube in her bladder (*Foley catheter*) to drain the urine and keep the bladder out of the way of the surgery we were about to undertake. We placed cloth towels around the lower portion of the patient's abdomen and then clipped them together with special instruments. We then placed clean sterile sheets on top. Using a sterile purple marking pen, Dan drew a curved line across the patient's abdomen a few inches above her pubic bone.

"Ok, let's test to be sure she is numb from the spinal," he instructed me.

I pinched the skin on both sides of the purple line with a toothed instrument. No reaction by the patient; the spinal was working.

"Now take the scalpel and follow that line I drew," Dr. Folger said. I grasped the knife like a pencil and followed the line. A thin white line appeared as I tenuously barely nicked the skin.

"Not like that," came his instruction. "Put your index finger on top of the handle and use the belly of the blade. Bear down a bit." On the second pass, I cut completely through the skin and a small amount of fat prolapsed through the *Pfannenstiel incision* (a crossways skin incision on the lower body).

"Ok now incise the white fascia in the middle with the second *deep knife* (the first scalpel is not used here for fear of contaminating the wound with skin bacteria)."

We then extended the fascial incision both ways with scissors. The *peritoneum* was next—a thin glistening layer below the fascia. This was easy to incise. Next came placement of the large metal bladder blade to hold everything out of the way. And now we were looking at the pregnant uterus. The uterus is one of the most miraculous organs in the human body. It starts out the size of a small pear, expands over the course of pregnancy to contain an eight-pound human being, a placenta, and two quarts of amniotic fluid. Almost one-third of the blood being pumped by the pregnant patient's heart is routed through the uterus to supply oxygen and nutrients to the growing fetus. Then at the end of the pregnancy, we take out the baby and the placenta and tell this amazing organ to contract immediately to stop the bleeding from where the placenta was once attached just a few moments earlier. And sometimes later in a woman's life—we ask it to do it all again!

We carefully made a small incision in the lower part of the uterus and then used special scissors to extend the incision to the left and right. The bag of amniotic fluid bulged through the incision. Dr. Folger grabbed an instrument and broke it.

"Now reach down with your hand, flex the baby's head, and then bring it up into the incision," he instructed me. After the baby's head was peeping out of the incision, we sucked the fluid from the baby's mouth and nose with a rubber bulb device and then handed him to the circulating nurse.

"Now reach in and create a plane between the placenta and the uterine wall and pull out the placenta," Dr. Folger said. The placenta came out easily. And then there was blood everywhere. I have scrubbed with general surgeons at some C-sections when there is the possibility of unexpected complications. They are always amazed at the amount of bleeding that takes place after a baby is delivered by C-section.

"This is more than I've seen in any trauma patient," they would often remark. "Yes, but the good Lord knew we obstetricians would be sloppy surgeons at this operation. He gave every pregnant woman about two extra pints of blood to prevent problems," I would respond.

"Start the Pitocin," Dr. Folger told the anesthesiologist.

"Go ahead and massage the uterus," he told me. Miraculously, the uterus contracted down and the red sea parted. We closed the uterine muscle in two layers using *cat gut suture* (the suture is actually made from sheep intestines). Then we proceeded to reverse the steps we had used to get to the uterus, closing each successive body layer with its own suture. Finally, we closed the skin with stainless steel staples.

The case had taken more than the usual forty-five minutes to an hour for a *primary* (first time) C-section. We were approaching two hours. Dr. Folger's wife had recently delivered their first child earlier in that month. Later in the operation, the circulating operating room nurse had stepped out for a brief time and had now returned. The phone in the OR rang and she answered it.

"Ahuh, ahuh, just a minute," she replied into the phone. "Dr. Folger, this is your son calling. He was wondering if you could get this case done so you could make it to his college graduation," she said.

Dan turned three shades of red behind his surgical mask and glared at the nurse. This will be a long chief year he concluded.

We usually were allowed to leave the hospital around noon after a night of call once our hospital tasks were completed from the decisions made during the morning's rounds. On one particular day of call, I had admitted a twenty-year-old patient who was pregnant with her first baby. Unfortunately, she was a brittle diabetic and had presented to our hospital in *diabetic ketoacidosis*. In this condition, a low level of insulin results in extremely high blood levels of *glucose* (sugar). My patient's *glucose* level was near 2000 (normal is about 100). Because there is a lack of insulin in diabetes, the body starves because it needs insulin to use glucose as a fuel source. Acid is produced in the bloodstream and the high glucose also leads to extreme dehydration. To make matters worse, my patient's fetus, who was just three weeks from being due, had died in the womb from the derangements in my patient's system. We would need to slowly correct her metabolic condition while inducing labor at the same time. An internal medicine resident met with me and we developed a plan of care. I carefully administered the prescribed doses of insulin, fluids, and electrolytes. Each hour we drew blood samples for testing. My patient's condition improved gradually and her labor advanced. Towards midnight, she began to experience painful contractions and I ordered an epidural for pain relief. While I was attending to another patient, the anesthesiology resident administered a one-liter fluid bolus containing glucose (intravenous fluids without glucose are usually given before an epidural to prevent low blood pressure when the epidural is activated). Much to my dismay, my patient's next blood sugar level was back to where we had started when she first arrived! And so, we began the whole process again. After a long night, I headed out to the postpartum hospital unit at 6 a.m. for rounds.

When I came back to check on my patient at around noon, she pleaded with me, "You have taken such good care of me. Can you please stay and deliver my baby?"

'Sure," I said with an exhausted smile. Five hours later, I delivered a beautiful baby boy and placed it in his mom's arms as she wept. I set my alarm for 5 a.m. this time before I allowed myself to fall into bed that evening with my clothes still on.

During my fourth month on my OB rotation, I faced my first near-death experience of a pregnant patient. The patient was a young black, athletic woman who was pregnant for the second time. When I took her history, I learned that she was a long-distance runner for a local university. Her labor was fairly uncomplicated and her nurse moved her to the delivery room close to the midnight hour. The patient delivered her little daughter effortlessly after only two pushes and then, she fell unconscious.

"Call the second-year resident stat," I instructed the nurse. After all this was the most senior resident in the hospital and I was in uncharted territory. I also asked the nurse to call the OB faculty. In those days, the obstetrical faculty took call from home and rarely if ever came into the hospital. By the time the second-year resident arrived in the delivery room, the patient's blood pressure had fallen to an extremely low level—60/40 (normal would be about 100/60).

"Her left side is turning purple," the nurse pointed out. Sure enough, I noticed a purple color starting to become apparent on the patient's left flank.

What could this be? I thought.

I heard the nurse talking to the attending on the phone after she had reached him, "Dr. Bogs they need you now."

"What's the deal?" said the sleepy voice on the other end of the phone.

"You tell him to get the F... in here now," shouted the second-year resident.

We were prepping the patient's abdomen in order to do an exploratory surgery when Bogs came flying through the operating room door. His wedding ring caught on the door handle and cut into his ring finger causing him to bleed profusely. He donned a surgical gown and put on sterile gloves. I could see the blood inside his glove surrounding around the fourth digit of his left hand. The anesthesiologist quickly put the patient to sleep, and we made a vertical incision on her abdomen. Bright red blood welled up as we entered her *peritoneum* (the thin layer of tissue that surrounds the inside of a patient's abdominal cavity). Her entire abdomen was filled with blood! We inserted the suction to remove the blood but more appeared as fast as we removed it. We resorted to using our hands to spoon the blood over the sides of the surgical incision.

Still unable to see the source of bleeding, Fred told the circulating nurse, "Call down to the emergency room and see if we can get a general surgeon up her to give us a hand."

A second-year surgery resident arrived from the emergency room with a metal handle in his hand.

"Here, place this on top of the *aorta* (the main blood vessel from the heart to the lower part of the body) and press down," he instructed. The red sea parted. We could see that the blood was coming from a tear in the artery that supplied the patient's left kidney. An *aneurysm* (an out pocketing of the vessel from a congenital weakness) had ruptured when my patient was pushing to deliver. Bogs placed a clamp across the vessel as the anesthesiologist frantically tried to keep up with the blood loss by administering unit after unit of red blood cells. The general surgeon attending soon arrived from home.

Peering over the incision he asked, "Whatcha got there? Looks like a renal artery aneurysm. Damn we're going to lose a good kidney. Too bad you guys didn't use a vascular clamp on that vessel." All of us looked up at him from the table. We all just wanted to respond with a, "Really!"

I noticed that there appeared to be a cast on the surgeon's right arm. Now what good was he going to be to us?

"Give me a minute, it's a minor break of my radius. I'll take the splint off and scrub", he instructed. He soon appeared in the operating room gowned and gloved. Ten minutes later a "good kidney" left my patient's body and appeared in the specimen tray. Her blood pressure had now returned to the normal range. My patient would survive.

The following Monday morning rolled around and I accompanied the other three residents on the obstetrical service at the university hospital to the usual conference room where we met every morning at 8 a.m. for morning report. This was a daily occurrence— all of the patients were presented to the OB attending physician and the *chief resident* (the fourth-year resident on the service). A plan of a care was developed for the new patients and management plans for ongoing patients were updated. Dr. Bogs was our attending that week. After we had finished going through all the patients, Bogs spoke, "I guess everyone has heard what transpired on Friday night with the patient that had a renal artery *aneurysm*. Thank god we had the help we needed to deal with it. I think this case illustrates why I am going to ask the chief residents to begin to sleep in house each night. We are seeing some complex patients sent in from all over our state."

Tom, the senior resident on the OB service protested "The chief resident has never slept in before. This is unheard of! We are going to take this to the program Director and the Chairman."

Up until now the in-house OB service had been run at night by interns with supervision by second- and third-year residents. When the new resident team took over the obstetrical service at the beginning of the following month, a new rule was now in place—the chief residents were now required to take turns sleeping in the hospital house every sixth night. This was a major change to the resident coverage. I could no longer look forward to my senior year of residency with no in-house call. Fifteen years later in my career, changes in residency rules would require me to sleep in the hospital as the supervising attending physician.

In our intern year, our rotation on general surgery took place at the inner-city hospital. The hospital served the less fortunate of the city and was staffed predominantly by residents from the university program, with only a few attending faculty for supervision. The inpatient surgical service was run by the chief resident. A third-year surgical resident and two interns made up the remainder of the team. We were responsible for all the elective surgeries that came from the outpatient surgical clinic—mainly inguinal hernias. The bulk of the service however consisted of admissions from the emergency room, many of whom were victims of trauma. The interns on the service were considered the "grunts." We changed dressings, wrote daily progress notes in the chart, and occasionally were allowed to actually suture a wound close at the end of a surgical case.

On one particular day, our team was called to the emergency room to admit a patient with a rectal obstruction. When the surgery team arrived to the ER, the surgery intern assigned there presented the case to our group.

"He was playing with this electronic device when he pushed it up too far into his rectum and the thing got away from him," he said. He took us over to the X-ray view box where the patient's pelvic Xray film was displayed. Yep, a vibrator. One could make out all the internal components—the battery and the adjacent motor. And the craziest part was the thing was still running because the image was blurry from the movement.

The chief resident arrived. "Looks like he will need an *exploratory laparotomy* (an operation where the abdomen is opened with a large surgical incision) and a *colostomy* to remove this thing," he instructed. "Prep him and let's get him up to the operating room."

And then a thought came to me. "Mind if I try something before we cut this guy open," I said.

"Have at it," the chief replied.

I approached the embarrassed patient and asked his permission to try to remove the vibrator from below.

"Anything to keep me from having my belly cut open doc," he replied.

"Ok, I need you to get on your knees and push your butt up into the air," I instructed him. I went over to the gynecology room and retrieved the largest *speculum* (that's the metal duck bill–looking device that gynecologists use in the vagina to see the cervix to perform a pap smear). I also grabbed a "ring forceps."

"Now this may smart a bit," I cautioned my patient. With that I inserted the lubricated speculum into his rectum and opened the blades as wide as they would go. With the aid of a penlight, I could just see the bottom of the vibrator at the uppermost end of the speculum. I grabbed it with the ring forceps and slowed began to extract it. As it began to appear, an outer membrane appeared to be sliding off the device.

"Damn it. I think you're pulling off his *rectal mucosa* (the lining of the large intestines)," said the chief resident.

"I don't think that's possible," I replied. With the vibrator now totally removed, I looked it over. "It's a ribbed condom on the outside," I said. I hit the off button on the device, washed it in the sink, and returned it to the thankful patient. He left the emergency room smiling. The next day on rounds I was given the new title of the "speculum king."

Now known as "half speculum will travel," I was soon faced with another case where my gynecologic skills would benefit a male patient. The patient was an eighty-year-old frail-looking man who had been admitted for bright red bleeding from the rectum. A *sigmoidoscopy* (a short lighted scope that is inserted into the rectum) had failed to reveal the source of the bleeding. An *arteriogram* (an injection of dye that fills the arteries) had suggested the bleeding was coming from the *transverse colon* (the middle part of the large intestines). Our team took the patient to surgery and a large part of his colon was removed in order to stop the bleeding. After returning the patient to the surgical intensive care unit, I was called emergently to the bedside. My patient had begun to bleed again. I arrived to find him sitting in a pool of blood.

"Can I have you get on your knees?" I instructed my patient. I asked the nurse to retrieve a vaginal speculum. She looked at me bewildered.

"To do what?" she said.

"You'll see," I responded. I placed the device into the patient's rectum and opened the blades (not quite as wide as I had done in my previous male patient). There on the side wall of the rectum about three inches up was a tiny blood vessel pumping bright red blood. A careful placement of a simple stich and the bleeding stopped. This had been the source the entire time! The surgery team had come to decide that having an OB-GYN on the team had its advantages.

It was now June of my intern year and I was on my last two-month rotation on the OB service at the university hospital. Even though I was feeling more confident as a physician, as I neared the end of my internship, I would continue to be humbled by new patient experiences.

The nurse came to get me one day when I was staffing Labor and Delivery.

"I need your help," she said. "I am not sure how to handle this situation. My patient is in active labor and in quite a bit of pain. Her husband tells me they are using the Bradley method of natural child-birth. She really wants an epidural but he told me that is not what she really needs."

As I entered the room, I was greeted by wails of pain from the patient. She looked at me through tears in her eyes, "Please, Dr. Moise. I can't take this. I need an epidural."

Her husband was standing at the bedside holding his wife's hand. "We've talked about this in our Bradley classes. I'm her coach. She really doesn't want an epidural."

The patient interrupted this statement with another wail of pain with the next labor contraction, "Please, give me an epidural."

"No sweetheart, we talked about this, you're doing fine," her husband responded. "You really don't need an epidural. I'm not going to let you fail and give in to this pain."

"Sir, I'm going to get the anesthesiologist," I responded. "Your wife is in early labor and we have aways to go before she delivers this baby."

"No, this is not what she wants," came his answer.

"I'm sorry but we are going to move forward with this," I said. "Your wife is my patient; you're not. I am here to take care of her. She will get an epidural. If you refuse to let me do this, I will have security escort you to the waiting room and you WILL miss the delivery of your son."

Dejected, the patient's husband sat down in the rocking chair next to the bed. I returned to the room an hour later. The patient was smiling while the fetal monitor showed active labor contractions every three minutes.

"Thank you, thank you!" she said grasping my hand in a firm grip with tears in her eyes.

I looked over to her husband. "You were right to intervene. Thank you," he said.

Methods for relieving the pain of labor have changed dramatically over time. Initially all childbirth was "natural" with no real options for pain relief. As deliveries moved into a hospital setting at the turn of the century, obstetricians began to use narcotics for pain relief. The drawbacks however include extreme maternal sedation and even newborn depression due to the transfer of the medications across the placenta. In the 1950s, a French obstetrician introduced the *Lamaze* method of birthing[14]. This emphasized special breathing exercises to reduce the pain. Around this same time, an American obstetrician introduced the *Bradley* method of natural childbirth which emphasized the importance of the patient's husband as a coach[15]. In the 1970s, *epidural anesthesia* was introduced[16]. In this method, the patient's back is first injected with a local anesthetic. A large needle is then inserted into the back at about the level of the hip bones. Once the needle is located in the epidural space just outside of the spinal canal, a plastic tube is introduced and the needle removed. The tube is then taped in place. An injection of a local anesthetic agent then blocks the pain nerves in the lower part of the body. Unfortunately, the medication can also block the *motor* nerves in the same area, causing the patient to lose muscle control of their legs. Today, much lower doses of anesthetic medication are used often in combination with the injection of narcotics. A continuous infusion pump allows for a more even administration of the medications. These changes have resulted in an epidural method with less loss of motor function. Some of these methods have even been advocated as *walking epidurals*—the patient can actually walk to the bathroom with the epidural in place. More importantly, epidurals are not associated with sedation of the pregnant patient or her newborns. Mothers are now alert and can participate more readily in the birthing process. The procedure has become so acceptable that a recent study in 2019 found that 76% of women in labor in the USA received an epidural or spinal for pain relief[17].

Other curve balls would come my way during this first year. On the first day of my internship, my class of six residents all went to the *GME* office at the medical school to have our mug shots taken for our ID badges. We were never really instructed to wear our IDs, so the badges were often relegated to a pocket of a white coat or a locker. It was early in the summer towards the end of my intern year and the usual medical student clinical rotations on the obstetrical service had ended.

A medical student appeared on Labor and Delivery and introduced himself to me. "Hi, I'm Frank," he said. "I am really thinking about going into OB so I thought I would spend some extra time on Labor and Delivery if that's OK. Can I shadow you?"

At this point in my training, I had delivered more than my fair share of normal babies so why not let Frank do a few. With my guidance, he and I scrubbed together and I let him do six vaginal deliveries over the next few weeks. Then Frank disappeared. I figured he had gained the experience he wanted and was headed out to enjoy what remained of his summer before resuming classes in medical school. About a week later, the GME office sent us an edict—we would be required to wear our ID badges at all times. It seemed that an imposter had been working on various clinical services in our hospital stating that he was a medical student who wanted to "gain some extra experience." This individual had approached a pharmaceutical rep for some sample antibiotics. The rep not recognizing him, looked him up in the medical school directory only to find that he did not exist. He notified the GME office. "Frank" was found in the operating room holding retractors on an open-heart surgery case that day. He was ushered out of the hospital by security.

6

On My Own—Moonlighting

After I completed medical school and passed my certification exam, I was given a medical license from the state in which I was born. Unlike the law profession, which allows you to practice in several states if you make a certain grade on the bar exam, in medicine, each state has its own licensing requirements. The middle south state where I had just completed by OB-GYN internship only required completion of the first year of clinical training to issue a medical license. They of course go through a process of checking in with other states where an individual is licensed to be sure that one is in good standing. Given that I had never actually practiced in my native state, this cross check was easy. So, I applied for my second state medical license and it was granted to me on short order. This meant I could moonlight in outside hospitals to improve my dismal income from my OB-GYN residency. My intern year had also provided me with the skill and confidence to handle most acute situations in medicine. Since I was single at the time, a free weekend from call at the teaching hospital would mean extra dollars in the bank. To make life a little easier, the call schedule for the next three years of my training would be easier than my intern year. One of the senior OB-GYN residents had set up a system where we could take turns working in a nearby small rural emergency room for the weekend. We would arrive on Friday night and stay in a vacant patient room until Sunday evening. Meals were provide by the hospital as a perk from the menu the patients used. Our sleep was often interrupted with each new patient arrival to the ER; however, the patient load never amounted to more than ten patients per weekend. This meant an extra $800 in the bank for these forty-eight hours of work.

On one particularly slow Saturday evening, I was called to the emergency room to see a middle-aged man who had been in an auto accident. The emergency medical technicians had brought the man in by ambulance. He was lying on a wooden backboard with a plastic neck brace around his neck.

"Any pain anywhere," I asked.

"Nope, Doc, I'm OK," my patient responded. "Ready to go home. This was a fender bender. Not sure why we need all this stuff."

"Well it's just routine," I replied. "Let's shoot a few films."

At this small rural hospital, my next task was to call in the radiology technician to get the X-rays. I would need to read them myself as there was no radiologist on call. Thirty minutes later my patient was in X-ray for a *C-spine series* (X-rays of the neck spine). I looked over the images and they looked fine to me.

"Hmm, I seem to be missing one standard image," I said to the tech. When I worked in the emergency room in my intern year, I had seen multiple patients brought in after automobile accidents. The drill was the same for all of them. Get the films, review them to be sure there were no fractures that would indicate an unstable neck, and then if all was OK, remove the cervical collar. But something was missing. Then I remembered—the *odontoid view*. This is where the patient is asked to open their mouth and an X-ray is taken to make sure the *odontoid process* of the second *cervical vertebra* is intact (turns out the odontoid process is fairly important—it keeps our head from spinning around like an owl's). If it is broken one can transect the spinal cord and then you are paralyzed for life!

The tech responded, "Oh yeah, I forgot to get that one. I just finished school last year and we don't do many C-spine series here. I'll shoot it now."

I looked at the film—a total fracture. I ran to the stretcher in the ER and began to tape the patient's head down to the wooden back board with three-inch silk tape. Two pieces over the forehead, one across the chin and one under the chin.

I placed a call to my university hospital—"sending you a neck fracture," I told the orthopedic resident. Back into the ambulance went my patient for the sixty-mile ride to the city. I did not sleep well that night—I could have missed this!

Monday morning rolled around and I had pretty much forgotten about my near miss episode. I was walking in the corridor when I heard a shout.

A voice called out, "Hey, Doc, good to see you again. Look what they did to me." There was my patient walking towards me. Connected to his shoulders and fixed to his head with large bolts that penetrated the skin of his skull at four different points was the *halo* apparatus that is used for stabilize neck fractures. A close call!

The small rural hospital where our group of residents moonlighted knew that we were up-to-date on the most modern of treatments. When I was on the medicine service as an intern, we were beginning to use *tissue plasminogen activator (TPA)* in patients with *acute myocardial infarctions (MI,* or heart attack). This "clot buster" medication dissolves the clot in the small *coronary vessels* (the small blood vessels that supply oxygen to the heart itself) and allows blood flow to return to the dying muscle of the heart. This allows the damaged muscle to recover instead of scarring down. At the time, this therapy was new. Today, cardiologists prefer to place a catheter into the heart through the *femoral artery* (the big artery in the groin) and open up a tiny balloon in the blocked coronary artery (*angioplasty*). At the small rural hospital where I moonlighted, they were not familiar with TPA being used in MI patients. So, one weekend, I called the hospital administrator and told him that we really should stock at least one dose for our country emergency department.

Several months later, an ambulance arrived with a fifty-five-year-old gentleman with acute chest pain. Mr. Davis had been raking leaves on that fall day when he began to experience pain in his left arm radiating to his chest.

"Still hurts real bad, Doc," he told me as he lay on the stretcher. His stat EKG showed abnormalities consistent with an anterolateral MI. This was consistent with partial occlusion of the *left anterior descending coronary artery*—what is called the *widow maker* for its propensity to be associated with sudden cardiac death. Within thirty minutes, I had the pharmacist mixing up the TPA and it was being infused into Mr. Davis's IV in his arm. I called one of my fellow residents on the cardiology service at the university hospital and we decided to it would be best to transport my patient by helicopter.

Our rural hospital did not have a heliport, so I called the nursing supervisor. "Can I get all the cars moved from the ER parking lot. We are going to have a transport helicopter landing here in about thirty minutes," I requested.

Someone must have leaked the news to the rest of the hospital. A large group of nurses, housekeepers, and receptionists assembled to watch the university helicopter descend from the sky. We loaded Mr. Davis onto the transport stretcher and put him through the back door of the helicopter. Away it flew to the cheers of the onlookers. Several days later I checked on Mr. Davis in the *CCU (cardiac care unit)* at my university hospital. He had undergone an *angioplasty* soon after his arrival and was doing well.

When I was moonlighting in the ER, I obviously felt most comfortable seeing the pregnant patients that came in. This rural hospital had a small Labor and Delivery Unit that only did about ten to fifteen deliveries each month. They rarely saw anything like the complicated pregnant women that were transported to our university OB service from around the state.

One afternoon, the ER nurse called me from my room to see a pregnant woman reported to be about 30 weeks gestation (term pregnancy is 40 weeks gestation). Mrs. Schneider was a lovely young woman, but she appeared to be somewhat distressed.

"What brings you to the ER today," I inquired.

"I am having the worse headache of my life. I tried two Tylenol and that didn't touch it," she replied.

"Any other symptoms?" I asked.

"Every now and then I've been seeing some flashing lights since I woke up this morning," she replied.

Her BP was 140/100, a bit high. I asked the nurse to check her urine for protein with an indicator stick. It returned with a three plus result—also high. I now knew this patient was presenting with pre-eclampsia. The disease is called *pre-eclampsia* because if left untreated it can progress to *eclampsia*. *Eclampsia* is heralded by seizures and is one of the leading causes of maternal death in our country. The cause of *pre-eclampsia* remains unknown, although it is thought to be related to problems with the way the placenta implants into the mother's uterus early in the pregnancy. In any event, my patient had severe *pre-eclampsia*. More importantly, the headache and visual changes indicated a spasm of the blood vessels in her brain. Seizure and even bleeding into the brain could follow quickly.

I asked the nurse to call the pharmacy and have them prepare a six-gram loading dose of *magnesium sulfate*—a special intravenous salt used to prevent seizures in pre-eclamptic patients. I then called the university hospital to arrange transport since the patient was still premature and delivery was probably needed (the only real cure for *pre-eclampsia*). The baby would need to be admitted to the neonatal intensive care unit.

The pharmacy called back a few minutes later. "We have only one gram of magnesium sulfate in the hospital; will that do?"

"Not a chance, "I responded. "Where can we get the other five grams I need?" I knew the ambulance ride alone could stress my patient and precipitate seizures. An ambulance on an interstate was the not the best place to treat seizures.

There was an ambulance parked in the bay outside of our hospital. "If I find a nearby hospital that has what I need, can you go get it for me?" I asked the driver.

"Sure doc, tell me where to go," he responded. The nursing supervisor located the additional vials of magnesium at another hospital thirty miles away. Our ambulance left, lights flashing and siren blaring. While I waited, I thought it best to go ahead and give the one gram of magnesium I had. An hour later, the ambulance returned with the additional doses. After we infused it into my patient's vein, we loaded her into the very same ambulance and sent her on her way to the university hospital. She arrived to their Labor and Delivery

Unit without seizing and was delivered by C-section by one of my co-OB-GYN residents later that same day.

During the next three years of my residency, I continued to moonlight at two different rural hospital emergency rooms. Although most of us did this predominately for the extra money we could make, I felt we made a real difference in the care these patients received. Many of the country docs that staffed these hospitals were older and were not familiar with the rapidly changing practices of medicine. Some of my fondest memories in my career come from the appreciation those country patients expressed when I saw them in the worse of circumstances.

7

First Responder: OB-GYN Rotations at a Private Hospital

My second year of residency was much more humane than the intern year. One of our second-year rotations took place at a private hospital in the city. Our primary responsibility was to gain experience in gynecologic surgery but as a courtesy we did cursory history and physicals for all obstetrical patients admitted to the Labor and Delivery Unit. The private attendings would then manage the patients in labor with the aid of the seasoned obstetrical nurses.

On one particular night when I was on call, I received an urgent page for *fetal distress* by the Labor and Delivery nurse. This was an unusual night—this was the only patient *on the board*—the dry erase board that used to grace all Labor and Delivery units and displays the names, important demographics, and status of all the laboring patients. Since there was only one patient laboring on the Labor and Delivery Unit, there were no private attendings drinking coffee in the doctors' lounge waiting for other patients to deliver. I was the sole obstetrician in the hospital! I had met the patient several hours earlier and a quick history led me to discover that this was her third baby with two previous uneventful vaginal deliveries. Her labor had progressed and she was now completely dilated. The fetal monitor showed that her baby's heart rate had dropped down to the 60s for about three minutes (a normal fetal heart rate is 120 beats/minute). I told the patient's nurse to *stat* page the private attending and to tell her that I was taking her patient to the delivery room. There we re-assessed the heart rate—still in the sixties.

"Let me have a pair of forceps," I told the scrub tech. After placing the drapes on the patient's legs, I proceeded to place the first *blade* (one of a pair that makes up the instrument known as *forceps*). Part of the handle of the blade disappeared into the patient's vagina indicating that the head of the baby was still too high in the birth canal to do a safe forceps delivery. I decided to abandon the attempt at a forceps delivery.

"Ok, let's try a *vacuum*," I instructed the scrub tech. The *vacuum* is just what it sounds like—a soft plastic cup attached to a handle. It is attached to the baby's head and with the aid of a vacuum pump, one pulls on the handle.

With the first pull, there was no movement of the head. "Ok, let's move to a C-section," I instructed the OR personnel. It felt like an hour had passed since I was first called to the bedside! In reality, only ten minutes had transpired. The anesthesiologist proceeded to put the patient to sleep. Still no private attending in the hospital! Up until now in my training, I had always had an attending physician or senior resident across the operating table at C-sections assisting me to be sure that I was correctly performing the procedure. I was going to have to go this one alone for the very first time!

Normally, the obstetrician incises each layer carefully—skin, fascia, peritoneum, push the bladder down, then incise the uterus. But with all the adrenalin flowing in my system, I was looking at the head of the baby with one slice of the scalpel! *Had I cut the baby? No, thank god.* I quickly delivered a limp little body and gave her to the circulating nurse. She placed the little girl in the *warmer*—the little bed in the delivery room with overhead heat lamps where newborn babies are watched to see how they are making the transition to a new life.

I heard the nurse say, "No pulse."

"She can't be dead," I said. "We just had a heart beat five minutes ago!".

The anesthesiologist whisked over from the head of my baby's bed and quickly placed a breathing tube into the throat of her lifeless little body. He began to blow oxygen into the baby's lungs with a small inflated bag.

"Still no pulse," he exclaimed. "An *Apgar* score of zero at one minute." Virginia Apgar was an anesthesiologist who in 1952 came up with a scoring system for newborns at one and five minutes of life. The best score is a ten at each of the time points. A low score means the baby needs some form of resuscitation. My baby had a score of zero.

I placed a large gauze pack in the open uterine incision of my pregnant patient to stem the bleeding and then left the operating table to help with the baby at the warmer bed.

"Can you call the *neonatologist* (the high-risk pediatrician)?" I instructed.

"He is on his way in from home," the nurse responded. Me alone again! I had just completed by neonatal intensive care rotation at the end my intern year and I had attended several newborn *codes*.

"Ok, let's start chest compressions. Let me have a small feeding tube," I said. I immediately placed it into the large vein in the umbilical stump where this dying baby was only moments ago attached to its mother's lifeline. "OK let's guess the weight and tell me how much calcium and epinephrine to give?", I said to the neonatal nurse who had come from the high risk nursery to assist.

"She looks like about three kilos," said the nursery nurse. She quickly calculated some medication doses. I injected both drugs.

"We have a pulse," declared the nursery nurse within about a minute. At that moment, the cavalry arrived. The neonatology attending took over the care of the baby, later transferring her to the neonatal intensive care unit. The obstetrical attending finally arrived and scrubbed in with me to complete the C-section.

The next day I went to see the patient that had been the subject of my first solo C-section. "I want to thank you for saving my baby," she said as she hugged me.

Gynecologic surgery cases at the private hospital were the hallmark of our surgical experience for the OB-GYN residents in training. We typically scrubbed with a senior attending who let us do *our side of the case*. Again, the human body is almost a perfect mirror of itself. Most of the female organs have the same type of blood vessels coming from either side, thus requiring the same type of surgery to be performed on each side of the body. The on-call OB-GYN resident on this clinical rotation typically did the pre-operative initial history and physical for all the elective gynecologic cases so we rarely met these private patients until they were asleep in the operating room. Later in my career I would decide that this was poor medicine based on a personal experience with my daughter's surgery. The majority of cases were hysterectomies for various gynecologic problems—pain, bleeding, or *uterine prolapse* (where the tissue supports of the uterus are lost due to aging and the patient complains of pelvic pressure). Every now and then some unusual case came up.

On this particular day, I arrived to assist Dr. Stride with a *modified Coffey suspension*. No longer used in modern gynecologic surgery, the procedure was once employed for the treatment of a *retroverted* uterus (when the uterus is tilted backward in the pelvis). In our patient's case, this was thought to be the cause of painful intercourse. In this procedure, the *round ligaments* (two muscular structures on either side of the top of the uterus) are tied to the patient's *fascia* (that thick layer of abdominal tissue that holds us together) to tilt the uterus forward. Simple enough! Dr. Stride made a small two-inch incision on his side of the patient, fished around a bit to identify the round ligament on his side, and then sutured the structure to the anterior fascia.

"Now you do the same," he said to me. I mirrored his previous surgical moves and grasped the same round ligament structure and adeptly sutured it in place.

"All done," he said. "Simple."

Something bothered me, though I wasn't sure what it was. "Mind if I take a quick look," I asked.

"Sure", he replied. As I began to look at the structure that was sutured on the side opposite to me, I began to suspect it was not the round ligament. As I poked around, I realized it was the patient's *fallopian tube* instead! When I looked further on my side, I realized I had created the same error—the *fallopian tube* was sutured to the anterior abdominal wall. In essence we had performed a *tubal ligation* in this young woman (who on review of her history had yet to have a baby). We extended our incision and removed the sutures hoping there would be minimal damage to the fallopian tubes. In fact, both had been severed.

"This is awful. What should we do?" asked Stride. I had recently completed a clinical rotation at the university hospital on the infertility service. During that time, we assisted the attending surgeons in doing *tubal re-anastomoses*—a delicate procedure where the patient's tubes are repaired after a tubal ligation to allow them to conceive.

"I can try to put them back together if you want me to," I replied.

"Better you then me," he said.

I asked the nurse if there were any *surgical loops* (special glasses with magnifying lenses attached used by surgeons for precision work). She brought me a pair that were three times magnification from the cabinet where most of the surgeons stored their loops. I then asked for some 6-0 suture—a filament so thin that it is difficult to see well with the naked eye. Using the surgical method I had seen on my previous clinical rotation, I began to repair the patient's tubes. At one point, Dr. Stride asked if he could do his side. I had the nurse place the loops on his head and gave him the needle holder instrument. Stride was in his seventies and had that intentional tremor that eventually plagues all senior surgeons. After a few attempts at placing the first suture, he realized his limited dexterity was not going to allow for a successful repair.

"You take over, my boy," he said.

After the patient returned to the recovery room, I allowed Dr. Stride to describe to his patient what had happened and how we had attempted to repair the damage. We would be optimistic but would need to schedule a *hysterosalpingogram* (an X-ray test where dye is injected into the uterus to then spill into the fallopian tubes to check for their patency several months later). On a later clinical rotation at the private hospital, Dr. Stride ran into me in the hallway.

"Say that tubal repair you did for me a while back. Great job. The *hysterosalpingogram* looked normal." I sighed in relief.

There were four residents assigned to provide twenty-four-hour-a-day, seven days-a-week coverage at the private hospital for the month-long rotation. One of the senior residents suggested we each take a weekend of call in its entirety—Friday night through Monday morning. This would allow us to have three weekends off for the month. Made sense to me, so I agreed. After all this was the private hospital and elective gynecology surgeries as well as scheduled C-sections and inductions of labor were not done on the weekends by the private attendings. They valued their weekends off as well.

On my first weekend of call, things seemed relatively quiet. Around 10 p.m. on Friday night, a nurse paged me from the postoperative gynecology ward.

"I am concerned about Mrs. White," the nurse said. "She is Dr. Sloan's patient who underwent an abdominal hysterectomy on Wednesday for endometriosis. She did not have a bowel movement by today so Dr. Sloan ordered an enema. We gave her the enema at around 5 p.m.. She started complaining of pain about an hour later. I called Dr. Sloan and he asked if you could come see the patient."

"Be right up," I replied. When I arrived, Mrs. White complained only of some mild abdominal discomfort. She told me her pain seemed to get worse about an hour after her enema. Her vital signs were stable. On examination her belly was a bit distended but there was no real pain to palpation. When I listened with my stethoscope, I could hear bowel sounds.

"It's probably nothing," I told the patient. "But let's be safe and get a few X-rays of your belly."

The nurse asked me for the reason for ordering the test so she could call radiology with the request.

"Rule out perforation," I replied. "Oh and ask them to get a film of her upper abdomen with her sitting up so I can see her diaphragm," I said.

About an hour later I headed to radiology to look at the films. Some distended loops of large bowel were present. Nothing unusual for a patient with a *post-operative ileus* (a condition where the bowels are not working yet after surgery and the loops of bowel become dilated). I especially concentrated on the upright film—yep, no air under the diaphragm. If air was present, I would suspect a bowel perforation. I went back to see Mrs. White. She looked about the same. I called Dr. Sloan and gave him an update.

"I suggest we keep her *NPO* (nothing by mouth) for now and see what happens," I said. He agreed.

I instructed her nurse, "call me if her pain gets worse". An hour later, I was paged again.

"We need you to come see Mrs. White. She is complaining of worsening pain," her nurse instructed me. I arrived at the bedside shortly thereafter. Things had changed. Mrs. White's abdomen was now rock hard to my touch.

I called Dr. Sloan. "I think she has a perforation as a result of the enema," I told him.

"Well that would be unusual," he replied. Do you know how many times I have given my post-op patients enemas without any problems? And you said her films were negative for free air, right?" he replied.

"Right but her exam has really changed. I really think you should get a surgical consult and come see her," I said.

An hour later both Dr. Sloan and the general surgeon he consulted agreed that an *exploratory laparotomy* (a surgery where the abdomen is surgically opened to look for a problem) was indicated. I scrubbed in to assist with the surgery. As the surgeon open the perito-neum, the room filled with the odor of feces. Mrs. White's entire abdo-men was filled with the contents of her *colon* (large intestines). There in the lower portion of the *sigmoid* (the lowest part of the large intes-tines) was a small perforation. Apparently during the hysterectomy for endometriosis, Dr. Sloan had removed an endometriosis implant on this portion of the colon. This had probably caused a weakness in the wall. The pressure of the enema had resulted in a perforation at this site. The colon is filled with bacteria that are very virulent. When elective surgery is planned on the colon, a *bowel prep* is done. Lots of medications to stimulate bowel movements, diet restrictions, and even oral antibiotics are given in advance to minimize the risk for infection. However, in the case of the *unprepared colon*, the best course of action is to do a *colostomy*. The colon is transected and the open end brought out and sutured to the skin to drain into a special bag. The lower part of the colon is then sutured closed since it can drain in the usual fashion. If all goes well for the patient, the ends can be reconnected several months later. We proceeded to copiously irrigate Mrs. White's abdomen with liters of sterile fluid to remove as much of the feces as possible. We then performed the *colostomy*.

Things however, did not go well for Mrs. White. She was admit-ted to the intensive care unit and placed on powerful antibiotics in an attempt to ward off infection. I managed to make it to the call room at about 10 a.m. early Saturday morning after a sleepless Friday night. There was still almost forty-eight hours remaining for my weekend of call!

I was awakened from a deep slumber when my pager went off with a *stat* page—I was needed urgently in the intensive care unit. Running on pure adrenaline, I headed to the unit. The nurses pointed me to Mrs. White's cubicle. When I arrived, the nurse anesthetist had already placed a breathing tube and was *bagging* Mrs. White with 100% oxygen.

My first thought—where is the code team? "Please stat page the code team," I informed the nurses.

The four nurses surrounding my patient all looked at me with bewildered eyes, "Dr. you are the code team. What will you have us do?"

To say the least, I was a little caught off guard. At the university hospital, when a *code blue* is called on the overhead page, an entire team of residents, intensive care attendings, and anesthesiologists arrive to *run the code*. This is a skilled team that is called into action several times daily at a university hospital. It was true I had been involved with code situations when I was on the internal medicine service, but I had never really been called to be in charge and *run* a code.

But this was a small private hospital and I guess I was the best chance the patient had given the circumstances. So, I took my position at the foot of the bed and began to play the role of coach.

"Ok, let's get a back board under Mrs. White," I instructed. "Do we have a pulse?" I felt in the patient's groin and there was no evidence of a pulsating femoral artery. "Ok, let's start CPR", I said. Mrs. White had already been placed on a heart rate monitor as part of the routine protocol when she was admitted to the ICU. Her heart rate was now about forty from what I could tell. Now if the average person watches enough medical television shows, the next thing that appears in a code are the *paddles* to *shock* the patient.

"Stand back and be sure everyone is clear," is the usual line the actors use. But shocking a patient is only used to convert one type of heart rhythm that is ineffective in allowing the heart to pump effectively (usually *ventricular fibrillation* where the heart is just quivering) to another rhythm that allows the heart to work properly (*sinus rhythm*). My patient had *electro-mechanical disassociation*. This means the electrical system of the heart was trying to work but the heart muscle was not pumping. Shocking wouldn't help (despite what the TV actors say). So, we gave a series of standard code medications— *atropine* (to make the heart rate increase), *bicarbonate* (to correct the acid that was building up in the patient's blood), and calcium and epinephrine to get the heart to pump. After several rounds of meds, there was still no pulse. I was at a loss as to what to do. Mrs. White was in her late forties and it didn't seem right to give up yet.

"Let me have the epinephrine syringe," I said. Like FBI agent Goodspeed who administers an intracardiac injection of atropine in the movie *The Rock*, I decided to give the epinephrine directly into the Mrs. White's heart. What did I have to lose? I found a space between her ribs on the left front chest, plunged the needle halfway in, and injected the entire vial of epinephrine.

"We have a pulse," the nurse said. I looked up the heart rate monitor was beeping at 130. The patient's blood pressure was now 60/40.

"Let's start a *dopamine* drip now," I said. "And call her attending, I am exhausted!" Mrs. White held her own through Saturday night. However, on Sunday morning she was seen by the neurologist who declared her to be brain dead. The family elected to discontinue the ventilator and her heart stopped ten minutes later.

Fast-forward three years in my career—I had finished my OB-GYN residency and was only one week into a fellowship in *Maternal–Fetal Medicine* (high-risk obstetrics) when I receive a certified letter notifying me that I was being sued for malpractice. Apparently my very grateful OB patient whose baby I had "saved" was filing a lawsuit. My name was the first on the list of physicians being sued.

Depositions followed months later, but the case had not yet gone to court after five years. Unfortunately, the little girl died as a complication of the brain damage she experienced at the time of her delivery. The suit was settled for $20,000. $10,000 was paid on my behalf from my university hospital and $10,000 was paid by the private attending who was not in the hospital when the patient was in labor. My case was reported to the *National Practitioner Data Bank*. The other two patients from my memorable experience at the private hospital never filed a malpractice claim.

Medical malpractice is defined as an act or omission by a physician during the treatment of a patient that differs from the accepted practice in the medical community and causes injury to the patient. *"Primum non nocere* — First, to do no harm" is the basic tenet of medicine. No physician consciously inflicts harm on his/her patients.

At the start of medical school, all future physicians take the *Hippocratic Oath:*[18]

"I swear to fulfill, to the best of my ability and judgment, this covenant:

I will respect the hard-won scientific gains of those physicians in whose steps I walk, and gladly share such knowledge as is mine with those who are to follow.

I will apply, for the benefit of the sick, all measures [that] are required, avoiding those twin traps of overtreatment and therapeutic nihilism.

I will remember that there is art to medicine as well as science, and that warmth, sympathy, and understanding may outweigh the surgeon's knife or the chemist's drug.

I will not be ashamed to say "I know not," nor will I fail to call in my colleagues when the skills of another are needed for a patient's recovery.

I will respect the privacy of my patients, for their problems are not disclosed to me that the world may know. Most especially must I tread with care in matters of life and death. If it is given me to save a life, all thanks. But it may also be within my power to take a life; this awesome responsibility must be faced with great humbleness and awareness of my own frailty. Above all, I must not play at God.

I will remember that I do not treat a fever chart, a cancerous growth, but a sick human being, whose illness may affect the person's family and economic stability. My responsibility includes these related problems, if I am to care adequately for the sick.

I will prevent disease whenever I can, for prevention is preferable to cure.

I will remember that I remain a member of society, with special obligations to all my fellow human beings, those sound of mind and body as well as the infirm.

If I do not violate this oath, may I enjoy life and art, respected while I live and remembered with affection thereafter. May I always act so as to preserve the finest traditions of my calling and may I long experience the joy of healing those who seek my help."

Today, major advances in medicine allow once-incurable diseases to result in long-term survival—childhood leukemia, Hodgkin's lymphoma, HIV infection. Thus, patients have come to expect exceptional outcomes even in the most unusual of circumstances. The five most likely causes of malpractice claims include misdiagnosis, surgical errors, failure or delayed treatment, birth injury, and prescription errors. Medicine is an imperfect science— even the best mammogram can be read as negative by an experienced radiologist in a patient who develops metastatic breast cancer six months later (this is known as a *false-negative* test). It is not that the radiologist missed the lesion on the films. Instead, the cancer was too small or did not display the typical X-ray characteristics.

And then there is the all-important human factor—"to error is human." Doctors are not infallible. Finally, today's medicine involves a complex orchestration of human beings each with their own assigned task. Any one error in the system can result in a devastating outcome. Take a hypothetical patient who is admitted for an elective C-section at the end of her pregnancy. She will interact with the admissions clerk, the *phlebotomist* (who draws her pre-operative blood samples), the lab technician who runs her blood count, the blood bank technician who processes her type and screen test to be sure the correct blood is available, the admitting nurse who starts her IV, the admitting resident who does her history and physical, the anesthesiologist who places the spinal anesthetic, the central processing clerk that sterilizes the operating instruments, the team of the operating room circulating nurse, the scrub tech, the OB attending, and the OB resident who perform the procedure, the pediatric nurse that looks over the baby after he/she is born, the pediatrician who examines the baby the next morning, the recovery room nurse who looks after the patient immediately after her Cesarean section has been completed, the postpartum nurses, the medical assistant that checks the postpartum patient's vital signs ,and the discharge care coordinator (I have probably missed a few links).

Now what if our hypothetical patient has just experienced more than the usual blood loss during her scheduled C-section. After her blood count returns low on the day after the surgery, the attending physician orders two units of blood to be given. The postpartum nurse checks the patient's arm band with another nurse and confirms that the two identifiers on the patient's armband (usually the medi-

cal record number and the date of birth) match the label on the blood
bag. All checks out. About thirty minutes after the first unit of blood
is being infused, the patient complains of extreme back pain and her
urine turns dark red. A *transfusion reaction* is diagnosed and despite
corrective measures, the patient develops *renal* (kidney) failure and
must be on dialysis for three weeks. A *root cause analysis* investigation is later conducted at the hospital. This reveals that the phlebotomist mistakenly placed another patient's identifying label on the
patient's tube of blood that was drawn when she was first admitted.
This tube of blood was sent to the blood bank and was used to *cross-
match* the requested units of blood to be transfused. This resulted in
an incompatible unit of blood being administered to the patient and
the subsequent transfusion reaction.

Early in my career, I was taught to show my patient her labeled
tubes of amniotic fluid after I had performed a genetic *amniocentesis*
to check the chromosomes of an unborn baby. The objective was to
have her confirm her name and date of birth on the tube labels. In
earlier days, genetic *amniocentesis* was offered to all women who were
more than thirty-five years of age as they were labeled *advanced maternal age* since they were statically at higher risk to have a baby with
Down Syndrome. Today there are less risky blood tests that can look
for the baby's DNA in the pregnant patient's bloodstream (called *cell
free fetal DNA*) to accurately screen for *Down Syndrome* in all women.
When I was a fellow, a terrible case involving a serious error circu-
lated around in the local high-risk OB community. In some offices, ten
to fifteen patients might undergo an amniocentesis on a single day
to check for *Down Syndrome* in the fetus of these pregnant women.
Tubes of amniotic fluid would be stored in a central area for pickup
by the lab courier at the end of the day. On one particular day, the
office nurse was busy and left several tubes in the rack with patient
labels sitting nearby. For whatever reason, a pair of patient labels were

exchanged when they were placed on the tubes at the end of the day. When the results became available two weeks later, the first couple was informed that their unborn child had *Down Syndrome*. After much deliberation, the couple made the very difficult decision to abort their pregnancy. The couple with the second sample were told their unborn child was normal. Five months later, they gave birth to a little girl with *Down Syndrome*. Devastated, the couple elected to put this child up for adoption. So, in this case, one human error resulted in TWO devastating outcomes—the wrongful loss of a normal child and, in the eyes of the second couple, the wrongful birth of an affected child.

Of course, a single human error can affect a large number of patients as well. Take the case that occurred at a major health system on the East Coast. Technicians refurbishing elevators at one of the system's hospitals needed containers to store discarded hydraulic fluid. They secured empty detergent cannisters from the nearby surgical instrument processing center. The drums were later moved to the loading dock of the hospital, picked up by a health supply service, and then redistributed to two of the system's hospitals. Surgical instruments were processed with the "detergent" for two months. More than 3,000 patients underwent surgeries with these instruments. During this time, processing technicians noted that the instruments felt "oily" and continued to alert their supervisors. Finally, an investigation of the dishwashing equipment determined the error. The healthcare system settled with the affected patients for an undisclosed amount of money.

Patients sue when they feel they have been wronged. Often this is because their physician does not explain the error or fails to admit genuine regret. Some patients sue their physician to punish them for their error. Many patients file a suit to simply understand what went wrong.

Malpractice cases are civil cases and are not heard in criminal courts. Each state has its own set of statutes related to medical malpractice. There is often a *statute of limitations*—a two-year time period is common once the injury is discovered. This means that if an instrument is left in the patient at the time of surgery and it is not found until an X-ray is done three years later, the patient can still file a lawsuit. In some states, the *plaintiff's attorney* (the attorney for the patient) has to file a letter declaring an intent to file a lawsuit. This gives both parties an opportunity to *settle* a case before a lengthy legal process begins. Once a case is filed, both the *plaintiff* and *defense attorneys* will seek *medical expert witnesses*. Most states require that the *expert* be in active clinical practice; some require that they be licensed in the same state or an adjoining state where the alleged malpractice incident occurred. In addition, some states require that the medical expert be certified in the same area of medicine that involves the allegations of the case. A good *expert* reviews cases for both the plaintiff and defense. In other words, they review the facts of the case for its merit. However, this is often not the case. Many *experts* are dubbed *hired guns* reviewing only for the plaintiff and often rendering suspect opinions. The *expert's* job is to educate the attorneys on the aspects of medicine in the case and to pass judgment as to whether the *standard of care* has been met. In all of my years of *expert* review work, I have been amazed how quickly the average attorney can become knowledgeable about even the most complex of medical conditions. Defining the *standard of care* is a pivotal part of any malpractice case. Someone once said that "all politics are local." In fact, "all medical practice is local" as well. In some situations, there are clinical guidelines that have been published by various national organizations or *colleges* such as the American College of Obstetricians and Gynecologists. If the *plaintiff's expert* believes that the *standard of care* was violated, then the case may move forward to the *discovery phase*. Often written questions called *interrogatories* are sent by either party. These are usually followed by oral *depositions*. These sessions of oral testimony are taken under oath with a court reporter present to keep a written record. Having done multiple *depositions* in my career (mostly as an expert witness), I find them very entertaining. The lawyers for each side usually enter into boisterous arguments since there is no judge present to keep the peace. A favorite ploy is for the lawyer to state an objection for his/her client, "Already asked and answered," comes the objection. This flusters the questioning attorney who then tries to reword the question. Often this attempt is followed by another objection, "Already asked and answered." What amazes me is how adversarial the atmosphere can become. Then at the end of the deposition, the two attorneys will go have coffee together. I guess they are taught this decorum in law school. Perhaps they begin to learn it in debate club in high school.

In any event, physicians take the criticism of their medical care on a personal level. The malpractice allegations are insults to their integrity. Physicians don't have coffee with attorneys after they have weathered a deposition. Both the physician and the nurse caring for the patient are deposed first. Sometimes the patient herself and her partner are also deposed. Finally, the deposition of the experts for both sides of the case follows. At this point the case may settle or the plaintiff's attorney may decide to proceed to a jury trial. In a criminal case, the facts are weighed by the jury and a decision is made based on the concept of *beyond a reasonable doubt*. In a malpractice case, the concept guiding the jury's decision is *more likely than not* (i.e., there is a 51% chance). Plaintiff attorneys must weigh their chances for successful outcome for their client. Patients usually do not pay attorney fees upfront so the plaintiff attorney must pay the expenses of the expert witnesses. Typically, the plaintiff attorney will take a 30% share of any final financial outcome of the case.

There are three types of damages that result in financial judgements in medical malpractice cases—*general* (pain and suffering), *special* (future medical expenses; loss earnings), and *punitive* (a message from the jury that they believed the physician caused undue harm). Original attempts to curb outrageous jury awards included *no fault compensation programs* in such states as Florida and Virginia. In these states, obstetricians and hospitals pay annually into a plan that provides compensation for medical expenses for children who suffer a birth injury. Patients must be informed if the physician participates in the plan at the start of the pregnancy since their legal options will be limited if a birth injury occurs. Other states have set up medical review panels that decide the merits of the case before a formal lawsuit can be filed. Although the decision of the panel is non-binding, its conclusions are discoverable at the time of trial. Therefore, most plaintiff's attorneys will not move forward with a case if the panel finds that there was no deviation from the *standard of care*.

Finally, *tort reform* at the state level has probably had the greatest impact on medical malpractice. *Caps* (limits) on non-economic damages have now been instituted in more than 50% of the states. As an example, the state medical society in Texas pushed for major tort reform in 2003[19]. This was passed into law by the state legislature and signed by the governor. A cap on non-economic awards of $250,000 for all the physicians involved in the care of the patient was a key part of the reform. Hospitals were also capped at $250,000 per institution and $500,000 if more than one institution was involved. As a result, medical malpractice claims decreased by 57%, payouts decreased by 35%, and malpractice insurance premiums for Texas physicians plummeted by almost 50%[20]. Despite the assurance that tort reform would decrease the costs of "defensive medicine," no changes in total healthcare costs were noted in the state. But not every state has managed to adopt tort reform. The average OB-GYN in California pays $49,800 annually for medical malpractice premiums, while the same physician in Florida paid $205,400 in 2021[21].

8

In the Trenches—Training at the Inner City Hospital

In 1978, Samuel Shem published the classic *The House of God* describing his life experiences in his intern year during his internal medicine training. One of his main characters was "the fat man"—a senior resident that was all-knowing, who mentored the intern class on how to survive their first year in the hospital. My "fat man" was Dr. John Lang. He was always the life of the annual Christmas party. Often when he drank a little too much, he would sneak up the back stairs of our inner-city hospital and have the nurses start an IV and give him a "banana bag"—a bag of intravenous fluids with a vitamin mixture that made it yellow in color. John had a tradition—he would always call the new second-year resident on their first night of call at the inner-city hospital to pull off some sort of prank. This first call night was already intimidating enough for the second OB-GYN year resident in our program. They were the most senior residents in the entire hospital and responsible for all things related to any female patient with reproductive issues.

I did not escape John's prank. It was about 8 p.m. my first call night and everything was relatively quiet. There were only two patients in labor and they were doing well.

One of the Labor and Delivery nurses paged me to the unit. When I called back, she informed me, "There's an outside physician on the phone that wants to transfer an OB patient to our hospital."

"Ok, be right up," I responded. I answered the phone, "Sorry to make you wait sir. I had to come up from seeing a patient in the ER."

"No problem," came the voice from the other end of the phone. "Listen I am a family practice doctor here in Smithville and I need to send you this pregnant patient."

"Ok tell me about her," I replied.

"Well, she is about 30 weeks pregnant and she is having premature contractions. I checked her cervix and she is about four centimeters dilated. The funny thing is that I felt this rope-like structure in her vagina that seemed to have a heartbeat."

"Oh my God!" I exclaimed. "That is a prolapsed umbilical cord. She needs an emergency C-section."

There was a silence over the phone that seemed to last an eternity. "Hmm, I thought since she was so premature it would be better to go ahead and get her headed to your hospital. The ambulance left five minutes ago," came the response.

I thought to myself, "this cannot be happening to me on my first night of call here." "Well you'll just have to call the ambulance and have them turn around and come back to your hospital," I instructed him. "This baby is going to die!"

At that point, I heard a mysterious chuckle on the other end of the phone. "Ken, this is John. Gotcha. Welcome to your first night on call."

A few nights later, I was called by the nurses on Labor and Delivery to examine a patient who presented in labor with her second baby. The presenting fetal part did not feel hard like a head. It was soft and I my glove had *meconium* on it when I removed it from the vagina (meconium is the green slimy first bowel movement of a newborn baby). Everything said this was a *breech*—the patient would need to be delivered by C-section. I would have to call the third-year resident in from home to assist in the surgery. I wanted to be sure of the presentation, so I ordered a pelvic X-ray. I looked at the film—yep an *incomplete breech* (the fetus was presenting in a "sitting bull" position). I called the senior resident to come in.

"Go ahead and get the patient prepped and get the spinal in. I'll be right there," he said.

The nurses and I brought the patient from X-ray to the elevator and took her to the operating room. Our hospital did not have an anesthesiologist on call at night. There was only a nurse anesthetist to assist. For this reason, almost all of our C-sections at night were performed under *spinal anesthesia*. The OB resident would perform a spinal tap and inject a medication then lay the patient down. Ten minutes later, the patient would be numb from her breasts to her toes. We painted the patient's abdomen with *betadine*. The scrub nurse and I then covered the patient with sterile cloth drapes. The third-year resident arrived and scrubbed in. I made the incision in the skin, then in the facia. I then incised the uterine muscle carefully so as to not nick the buttocks of the baby.

The third-year resident peered into the incision, "Hmm, looks like a head to me."

I reached into the uterus and lifted the baby's head out then delivered the rest of the body. Everyone looked at me. I was the one that called for the C-section for breech.

"I swear I saw a breech on the X-ray," I responded to their glaring looks. After the case, I went to retrieve the X-ray—it was a breech presentation!

I went to the recovery room to talk with the patient. "Say, when you were riding the elevator to the operating room, did you notice anything unusual?" I asked.

"Now that you mention it, Doc, my baby really seemed to move a lot during that elevator ride." I was vindicated!

When we were on call, we covered both the OB patients and any GYN patients in the hospital as well as those that came to the ER. During one of my call nights, a sweet elderly patient arrived complaining of back pain. She has advanced cervical cancer and bilateral *nephrostomy tubes* were coming out of each side of her back. The left-sided tube did not appear to be draining. Patients with advanced cervical cancer develop blockage of the *ureters* (the tubes that connect the kidneys to the bladder). In some cases, a tube is placed through the patient's back into the kidney itself to allow it to drain above the blockage caused by the cancer. The placement of *nephrostomy tubes* in patients with advanced cervical cancer is controversial. The procedure will only prolong the patient's life for a short time. I decided that my patient's pain was probably related to a blockage of one of her nephrostomy tubes. I asked one of the senior general surgery residents what dye I might use to do an X-ray to see if the tube was patent. He told me *gastrograffin* would be his preference (I later learned that the correct dye was called *renografin*). Thinking that I would move ahead with a diagnostic procedure, I asked the night radiology technician if she would mind shooting the X-rays for me as I pushed the dye. She agreed. The dye went through the tube very easily indicating that it was draining. I admitted the patient and placed her on intravenous antibiotics, thinking the pain was probably now related to infection. The next morning, I learned we had used the wrong type of dye. The *gastrograffin* had solidified and was now blocking the entire tube. The nephrostomy tube would have to be replaced.

A few days later, I was called to my Chairman's office to discuss the incident. A long green couch was located just outside the academic office of the OB-GYN Chairman. When residents were called to meet with the Chairman, it was never to receive laudation for excellent patient care. Upon arrival, we were required to wait on the green couch. I was instructed by the secretary to enter Dr. Burns' office and to have a seat in the chair across from his desk.

Burns looked up at me after closing the chart on his desk. "Ken, I received a call from the radiology attending at the inner-city hospital. Since when do OB-GYN residents perform fluoroscopic procedures on their patients at night?" he asked.

I was not sure how to answer. "I guess I thought I was trying to help my patient. I overstepped by boundaries," I replied.

"Let this be a lesson for you. Next time wait until the following morning and consult the radiologist."

"Yes sir," I responded.

9

Choosing a Subspecialty—
Next Steps in Training

The Chairman of our OB-GYN department, Dr Burns, was "old school." Having come to our university from Johns Hopkins medical school, he declared Saturdays to be a work day until at least noon. Most medical school departments hold *grand rounds* on a weekly basis. Lectures on a variety of topics are provided by local or invited speakers from other medical schools. All residents and faculty attend. These lectures also provide an opportunity for local private physicians to hear the latest developments in their specialty. Grand rounds for our OB-GYN department were held on Saturday mornings. Attendance was mandatory.

Dr. Burns was a quiet man who showed little emotion. I remember on one occasion, all twenty-four OB-GYN residents asked for an audience with him regarding an issue that had developed with the attending physician that was assigned to supervise the residency training program. He came to the meeting and all four of the class representatives made their arguments as to why this individual should be replaced. At the conclusion of the meeting, Dr. Burns thanked us for our time, then left the room. The message was clear—the current residency director had his complete support and there would be no changes.

Our Chairman was always in his office by 5 a.m. each day. We knew this because the light in his office could easily be seen from the resident parking lot. The second-year resident on the oncology service at the university hospital usually arrived by 4 a.m. each day to get all the daily tasks completed before rounds. Morning rounds with the attendings on the service were at 6 a.m. Surgery cases always started at 7 a.m. sharp. It was rumored that Burns must have had a special key for the hospital elevator since the doors always opened and he stepped out precisely at 6 a.m. each day when he was on service. Most of our oncology patients were elderly and recovering from extensive surgeries. Often there was a *nasogastric (NG)* tube in their nose to empty their stomach of any fluids it might secrete while the patient's bowels were still recovering from an extensive surgery.

My chief instructed me early in the rotation, "Make sure all the NG tubes are whistling Dixie when Burns gets here for rounds."

What I later learned was that the small blue tube on the side of the main suction tube was where air was brought into the stomach so that any liquids could be removed by the suction apparatus connected to the main tube. When the air was being pulled in, the little blue tube would issue a whistling sound, indicating that the whole mechanism was working. Being a second year on the oncology rotation was one of the most trying rotations of our training program as an OB-GYN resident. This was well known among the resident staff. After all it was the Chairman's service. Karen, the Labor and Delivery nurse who I had begun dating at the time, knew this as well.

She decided to backpack with a girlfriend across Europe while I was on the oncology rotation.

I was on call one night and was sleeping in the resident call room. It happened to be on the same floor as the GYN oncology service. My pager went off at around 2 a.m. When I looked at the digital screen, it was a *stat* page to the nurses' station on the oncology floor. Wiping the sleep from my eyes, I decided it better to just go there instead of calling.

"What's up?" I asked arriving a minute later.

"Dr. Burns' patient in room 1230 is coding—she has stopped breathing," was the response.

I immediately sprinted to the room to find one of the night-shift nurses performing CPR on the patient. Mrs. Gail was one of our oncology patients. She has undergone major surgery two days earlier for ovarian cancer. The surgery had gone smoothly and her recovery up until that moment had been uneventful.

"Let's stop compressions for a minute and let me check a pulse," I instructed. I was easily able to find a pulse on the side of the patient's neck over the carotid artery. But she was clearly not breathing. The hospital code team had not arrived to the room yet.

"Open the crash cart and let me have the laryngoscope and a 7.0 endotracheal tube," I said. I placed the scope into Mrs. Gail's mouth and was able to see her vocal cords with ease. I passed the plastic tube into her windpipe and blew up the balloon at the end of the tube that keeps air from leaking around it. We then attached the tube to a special bag to provide breaths with 100% oxygen.

"Call the ICU for me and let's get her to a bed," I instructed.

A few minutes later we had moved the patient from her bed to a stretcher and were on the way to the ICU. Once we had stabilized the patient, I decided to call Dr. Burns. It was his patient, and I knew he would want to know about the incident.

"Dr. Burns, Mrs. Gail in 1230 coded in the last hour. We intubated her and she is doing well here in the ICU," I said.

"Do you think I should come in?" he asked.

"Well, I have already talked with the family and I think they are OK," I responded.

"I think I'll come in anyway," he replied.

About thirty minutes later, I looked up to see Dr. Burns at the door of the ICU room. He was dressed in a neatly pressed collared white shirt with a necktie. He had obviously shaved very quickly that morning. Multiple small razor cuts were visible on his face.

"How is she doing?" he asked.

"She's fine. May have been a reaction to too much morphine but she is sedated now," I answered.

He headed to the waiting room to talk with the patient's family. And this was the Chairman of my department!

Of course there are always those moments in your training that are emblazoned into memory. As the second-year resident on the oncology rotation, often you are relegated to more menial tasks. In this particular surgical case, the chief resident was scrubbed with Dr. Burns. This was a unique case—the patient was from a small rural town and she had neglected to seek medical attention for what appeared to be the rapid growth of her abdomen. At sixty-two years of age, pregnancy could not be the reason. When she finally arrived to the outpatient clinic, a CT scan was ordered which showed an ovarian mass the size of a watermelon (for some reason, OB-GYNs like to describe female organs like fruit—lemon, orange, grapefruit, etc.). Physicians, especially those at teaching institutions, like to record their unique cases. These make for interesting talks for their trainees. And then, as my wife once told me, clinical stories are a great way of making a teaching point. The size of the mass in this particular case made the current patient worthy of a photograph. Digital photography was not yet on the horizon. Burns' camera was a small Kodak with a U-shaped metal frame extending about four inches in front of the lenses. This allowed the user to center the image in the camera without leaning over the surgical field to look through the viewer. Of course, the point was not to "contaminate" the sterile surgical field while still capturing the picture.

Burns had delegated me as the photographer that day. After a brief instruction prior to the start of the case, I accepted my privileged role. The patient was intubated with general anesthesia and her abdomen opened to expose the massive-appearing left ovary.

"Ok, stand on a stool and get this picture," Burns instructed.

I leaned in a bit and struggled to center the large structure into the area of the metal frame. As I snapped the picture, the frame dislodged from its attachment at the bottom of the camera, falling into the patient's open abdomen.

There was a silence in the OR for what seemed like an eternity to me.

Then Burns spoke in a calm voice, "Is this patient already on antibiotics?"

Not knowing what should be my next move, I decided to reach over and remove the metal frame from the open wound. I turned around and left the OR.

Afterwards, no one talked about what had happened. I later found out that the photo had turned out great!

I had always enjoyed the surgical aspects of OB-GYN. But oncology was different. On occasion, one could "cure" an early-stage cervical cancer with a *radical hysterectomy*. But more often than not, the surgeries were palliative with little chance for extended survival. Ovarian cancer represented the worse of the diagnoses. Patients typically did not present with symptoms until the disease had progressed to spread throughout their abdomen. *Debulking* of the tumor was done at the first surgery followed by several rounds of chemotherapy. Then a *second look* operation was done to see if any cancer remained. Often it did. But it was the operation called *pelvic exenteration* that had me rethink my future in OB-GYN.

Mrs. Brown was diagnosed with cervical cancer when she was thirty-one years old. She was treated with standard radiation therapy with promising results. Now, however, four years later, the cancer had returned. She would need an extensive surgery called a complete *pelvic exenteration* if there was any chance for survival. This meant that her vagina, uterus, tubes, and ovaries would be removed along with her bladder and the lower part of her colon and rectum. She would now have bowel movements into a colostomy bag. Her urine would come out into a separate bag through another opening in her abdomen. Mrs. Brown's operation took fourteen hours and required one surgical team consisting of an attending and a resident working through a surgical incision in her abdomen. A second team, which included me, operated from below in her pelvis. When we finished, one could see the operating room lights streaming from the abdominal incision all the way through where her vagina once existed. An internal fat pad that is attached to the upper part of the large intestines called the *omentum* was sutured down like an apron to occupy the space of the missing organs in her pelvis. My job over the next two weeks was to take Mrs. Brown to the treatment room every morning to irrigate her incision from below to allow scar tissue to build up. Mrs. Brown remained in the hospital for a month before finally being discharged.

In the early 1970's, three subspecialties in Obstetrics and Gynecology were created—Gynecologic Oncology, Reproductive Endocrinology and Infertility, and Maternal–Fetal Medicine (MFM; high-risk obstetrics). A fourth subspecialty was added later—Female Pelvic Medicine and Reproductive Surgery. This pales in comparison to the number of subspecialties currently available in the other major fields of medicine: fourteen in surgery, twenty in pediatrics, and thirteen in internal medicine.

When I first started my residency, I thought I would aspire to be a general OB-GYN perhaps practicing in a small town similar to the one where I had moonlighted in emergency rooms. But the idea of sub-specialization somehow intrigued me. Based on my experiences on my second-year rotation, I knew oncology was not an option. I spent a one-month rotation on the infertility service predominantly looking at *post-coital tests*. In this situation, the couple has scheduled sexual intercourse in the morning. Then the woman comes into the clinic and has a sample of mucous taken from inside her cervix. Under the microscope, one looks for motile sperm indicating that the patient's mucous is "not hostile" to her partner's sperm. This subspecialty was not for me either.

When you ask a medical student why they pick a particular specialty, they usually recall an experience with a faculty role model that made a significant impression on them. Dr. Bogs was such a mentor for me. He was one of the early academic leaders in the field of Maternal–Fetal Medicine. He was a consummate teacher holding fetal monitoring "strip rounds" once weekly. There he taught us how to interpret the electronic fetal monitoring that virtually all pregnant patients undergo to assess the well-being of their fetus during the course of labor. Many skills cross medical specialties. All of us are taught to read a chest X-ray or assess an EKG for evidence of myocardial infarction. Fetal monitoring is unique—only obstetricians and MFMs are expert in its interpretation—an important skill when this is the only means of assessing the well-being of an unborn child facing the possible devastating consequences of a problematic course of labor and delivery.

Dr. Bogs taught us other aspects of medicine as well. We were making rounds together one day on his private patients who had already delivered their babies. He went into the first room, sat on the patient's bed, and made direct eye contact with her. "How are we doing today?" he asked. "Any problems?"

"Doing great," she responded. "Ready to go home tomorrow."

We left and went to the second patient's room. This time Bogs stood at the foot of the bed and asked the very same questions. Then he walked away.

"Go back and ask both patients how long I was in their rooms," he instructed me.

An hour later, I went into the first patient's room. "Can I ask you if you don't mind, how long was Dr. Bogs in your room this morning?" I asked.

"Hmm, at least twenty minutes," she responded (it had actually been only five minutes).

I went to see the second patient. "Do you recall how long Dr. Bogs was in your room this morning on rounds?"

"About five minutes," she responded. "He seemed like he was in such a hurry."

I later told Bogs about my findings.

"Yep, it's all in the body language, my boy," he replied. "And here is another tip. If you want to cut a visit short with an especially talkative patient, sitting on the bed allows you the opportunity to the stand when you want to conclude the visit. This sends the non-verbal message to the patient—we're finished." This is a lesson I have not forgotten to this day.

Bogs was also skilled as a clinician. He always seemed to know how to pick the right time in pregnancy to *induce* a patient. His private patients would be admitted to Labor and Delivery first thing in the morning. He would come over midday and "break the patient's waters" to accelerate labor. The patient would be delivered early that evening before supper.

"Now that's how I keep a busy practice and still manage to sleep most nights," he would tell me.

Most OB-GYN departments are organized into divisions based on sub-specialties with the Directors of each division reporting to the Chairman. Bogs was appointed as the Director of the Maternal–Fetal Medicine Division during my intern year. In this role, he was responsible for setting policy and overseeing difficult patient decisions.

I was a third-year resident at the university hospital when the nurses were called at around 7:30 a.m. one morning by a patient's husband.

"My wife is 18 weeks pregnant and she has just passed out on the floor of the bathroom and she is snoring," he said. "What should I do?"

"Call 911," the nurse replied.

Reba Schneider arrived to Labor and Delivery by ambulance twenty minutes later. Her breathing was labored and she was unresponsive. Her pupils remain fixed and dilated even when I shined a penlight into them. We decided to place a breathing tube to help her breathe. A few minutes later, we were wheeling her stretcher into the MRI unit. The images were horrifying—a large amount of blood was replacing almost half of one side of her brain. An abnormal connection present since birth between a vein and an artery in her brain called an *AV malformation*, had ruptured. Neurosurgery came to see her on Labor and Delivery.

"There really is no reason to operate," the neurosurgeon said. Neurology came by and performed a series of tests and declared her "brain dead." Her husband was devastated.

"What am I to do?" he asked as he sobbed looking at the patient's nurse. "This is our first baby. We have been trying to get pregnant for five years."

Dr. Bogs arrived to assess the situation. He and I brought the patient's husband into a small consultation room just outside of Labor and Delivery.

"I am really sorry about this," he said. "We are going to have to make some decisions though. We can let her go, if that is what you wish."

Through tears, the patient's husband responded, "But we really wanted this baby."

"There have been a few cases reported where a mom is kept alive until the baby is far enough along to be delivered in a healthy state. But this decision is entirely up to you," Bogs responded.

"Is that even possible?" he asked.

"We can try," Bogs replied.

We admitted the patient to the intensive care unit and placed her on a ventilator. A tube was placed down her nose into her stomach to provide liquid nutrition. After she reach 26 weeks of the pregnancy, OB nurses would see her daily to check the fetal heart rate to be sure the baby was still alive. Ultrasounds revealed the baby to be growing normally. At 36 weeks, Dr. Bogs performed an amniocentesis to check to see of the baby's lungs were mature. The test returned positive. The next day the patient was moved to Labor and Delivery.

Most of the nurses had grown attached to the patient during her prolonged hospitalization. As a result, emotions ran high that day. A C-section was performed and Reba's little girl came out crying as soon as she was born. The operation was completed and mom, baby, and dad were taken to the recovery room to be together. At the dad's request, the breathing tube was removed. A few minutes later, Reba was gone. Her legacy looked over at her mother never to feel the warmth of her maternal embrace.

In its infancy, the subspecialty of Maternal–Fetal Medicine concentrated on pregnancy complications in the mother. Ultrasound was a relatively new technology and so the fetus remained an hidden passenger who could not be seen except by an occasional X-ray. In cases of blood incompatibility between a pregnant patient and her partner, Rh antibodies can form, causing the fetus to become extremely anemic. Dr. Bogs was one of the few MFM specialists in the country who had been trained to perform a life-saving procedure on these fetuses in these situations—an *intrauterine transfusion*. Performed for the first time in New Zealand only fifteen years earlier, a small plastic tube was placed into the unborn baby's abdomen using X-ray guidance[22]. Red blood cells (the same blood type as the mother) were then injected through the tube correcting the fetal anemia. During my reproductive endocrinology clinical rotation, I heard that Dr. Bogs was scheduled to perform one of these procedures. I made myself conspicuously absent from the infertility clinic that morning. I headed over to the radiology suite. I watched Dr. Bogs first check the suspected position of the baby with his hands placed on the pregnant woman's abdomen. Then using the X-ray machine, he marked a spot where he thought it would be safe to insert the needle through the skin, the womb ,and then into the baby's abdomen. He measured how deep the needle would have to be advanced to reach its target. After injecting a local anesthetic into the patient's skin, he expertly advanced the largest needle I had ever seen into the fetus. With the X-ray machine running, he injected a small amount of dye and watched it spread over the loops of intestines inside the fetus.

"Looks like we are in the right place," he said.

Then he inserted a plastic tube through the needle. A second later, the needle was out. The nurse then attached a syringe of red blood cells to the end of the tube and slowly pushed in the blood. Dr. Bogs then removed the tube from the patient's abdomen.

"All done," he declared. "We'll see how your baby does. You may need another one of these in a few weeks," he told the patient. I watched him wink at me as he left the room. I decided this is what I wanted to do in medicine!

Several weeks later, I sat down with Bogs in his office to discuss my future.

"I loved what you did for that fetus the other day," I said.

"Ken, we have been impressed with you. We would love for you to stay here and do a fellowship with us in Maternal–Fetal Medicine." A computer screen was notably lacking from Dr. Bogs' desk.

"I hear the folks at Yale are using ultrasound to guide the needle for intrauterine transfusions instead of exposing the fetus to X-rays," I said.

"Yep, I heard the same," he replied. "But I hope to finish out my career in MFM without ever turning on a computer or an ultrasound machine."

I paused for a moment. I revered this man. He was the reason I was thinking about continuing with further subspecialty training in MFM. But I felt I could see changes on the horizon coming to the subspecialty.

"Dr. Bogs, I really think those tools are the future of our specialty. I hate to disappoint you, but I am going to have to look elsewhere for a fellowship."

Unlike, residency training positions, fellowship training assignments were not the subject of a computerized match (although this would change in the future). Karen (my future wife) and I headed out to California during my third year of residency for a bit of vacation combined with a postgraduate course in fetal monitoring. The course directors were Dr. Freed and Dr. Granite. They had co-authored the text used in the course which was filled with unique and challenging cases. Based on this experience, I decided to apply for the MFM fellowship at their California university. Karen was excited—a chance to move to California and rub elbows with the stars. What more could a girl from a small town in North Carolina ask for? I went through the usual personal interview process. Dr. Bogs knew Dr. Freed so I had an excellent letter of recommendation. MFM fellowships involved two additional years of training after OB-GYN residency at that time. Now they are three years in length. The first year at the California program would be spent assisting with "maternal transports"—sick pregnant patients sent from smaller hospitals to the larger urban hospital. I would have to ride the transport helicopter to retrieve these patients—not something I cherished given my extreme acrophobia. When I asked about training in ultrasound or critical care, I was told these were off service rotations to get exposure in these areas. Not optimal in my opinion, but the program and its two leading faculty had a national reputation. I shook hands on a position to start the following July.

About a month later, I was looking through one of my journals when I noted an advertisement for a MFM fellowship position at a private medical school in the southwest. I recognized one of the names on the advertisement as a clinical professor in infectious disease that I knew from my medical school. I decided to make the trip for an interview. What could it hurt? I put on a suit and waited in the hotel lobby for the MFM faculty who was supposed to meet me to start my interviews. Thirty minutes went by past the time we were scheduled to meet; then an hour. I decided to walk across the street to the private hospital and ask around.

When I finally found Labor and Delivery, I asked the clerk at the front desk, "Has anyone seen Dr. Bale?"

"He's in the doctors' lounge around the corner," she replied. I headed there to find an individual with snakeskin cowboy boots propped on the table in the middle of the room.

"I'm here for a MFM fellowship interview," I said.

"Damn, I was supposed to get you from the hotel," Bale responded. "Guess the time slipped away from me."

Bale had recently transferred over from a neighboring medical school in the city after a falling out with the new Chairman of OB-GYN. We chatted for a while. He was interested in critical care obstetrics and was planning to set up a maternal intensive care unit at the inner-city hospital. Next was an interview with Dr. Wood. To say the least, I found him to be one of the most intense individuals that I had met in my short medical career.

"We do our own ultrasounds here. No radiologist. Obstetrical ultrasound belongs in the hands of the MFM," Wood bragged. He informed me that he had the first sophisticated ultrasound machine in the city and it cost almost a quarter of a million dollars—I was impressed. He showed me a computer program that he and Dr. Detrie had developed written in DOS language (Microsoft Windows was not even in development yet) for keeping track of ultrasound patients and printing reports. Even more impressive!

Later in the day, I was taken to the inner-city hospital. This large southwestern city had only two hospitals to care for the underserved population. One was a general hospital for trauma and general medicine, while the second was predominately an obstetrical hospital. When I arrived, I was taken on a tour of the "green room" – a large open area with thirty stretchers filled with laboring pregnant women. Standing at the door, the spectacle looked like the railroad scene of the wounded soldiers from the movie *Gone with the Wind*. I later learned that more than 18,000 women delivered every year at this hospital. A bit overwhelming. But as I pondered this overwhelming number of deliveries, I realized that I only had to deal with the high-risk pregnant women. The routine cases could be cared for by the medical students and the residents. What a potential training ground! My interview with Dr. Joy of OB anesthesia, cinched the deal. I noticed a map on his wall with six U.S. states shaded with various colors.

"If you don't mind me asking, what does this map represent?" I asked.

"We do more deliveries at this one hospital than any one of those six states," he responded. This cinched the deal! I called Karen and told her I had changed my mine. We would not be moving to California; we would be moving to the heat and the humidity of the southwest. She was more than disappointed. On later reflection, this was probably one of the best decisions in my career. To this day, when I see Dr. Granite at various national conferences, he reminds me of the fellowship that could have been.

Physicians are generally at the peak of their knowledge base when they complete their residency training. They are then required to pass a written *board examination* in their specialty. In some specialties, including OB-GYN, a collection of patient cases cared for by the physician over the first year of their practice is then submitted as a *case list*. The physician then *sits their oral boards*. Most physicians seek out a review course to prepare. Oral boards are a harrowing experience where senior physicians in the same field question the applicant for three straight hours on their case list as well as other hypothetical patients. A pass means you are now *board certified*. A fail means two more tries then back to repeat part of the residency. About 85% of graduates pass the oral exam in OB-GYN the first time. The process of education does not end there. One then moves into a *maintenance of certification (MOC)* phase. In my case this required taking another written test every ten years. Today, the MOC in OB-GYN involves a yearly review of some fifty peer-reviewed articles selected by the American Board of Obstetrics and Gynecology (ABOG). One has then to answer questions online from these articles with an 85% pass rate.

To maintain a state medical license, most states require that a physician have a prescribed number of *continuing medical education (CME)* hours. These can be obtained by attending local conferences, reading certain articles, or arranging to combine a vacation trip with a CME course offered by a commercial educational organization. Truth be known, all of these requirements do not make you a good doctor.

I was once told that to be an expert in anything, one has to gain about ten thousand hours of experience. Venus Williams did not win grand slam tennis events only because she had raw talent (although this is probably a good place to start). Her father had her on the tennis court when she was only seven years old. Through the years, she developed muscle memory as to how to uniformly perform a forehand or backhand swing. One of my mentors pulled me aside one day when I was a new attending physician. I had spent the better part of the night watching my private OB patient make slow progress in the course of her labor. Her cervix ultimately dilated to ten centimeters (also called *complete)*. But after three hours of pushing, the baby's head would not descend into the pelvis so we had to perform a C-section for the diagnosis of *cephalopelvic disproportion* (the baby's head was too big to fit though the pregnant patient's pelvis). It was 6 a.m. when Bill came through Labor and Delivery to make his usual morning rounds. I had just completed my C-section and I am sure I looked just like I felt—utterly disappointed and exhausted.

"I would have thrown in the towel probably around 2 a.m. I looked at her labor curve. She wasn't going to make a vaginal delivery with that first baby. I would have at least gotten three hours of sleep," he said.

"Bill, how could you be sure that was going to be the outcome? I wanted to give her every chance for a vaginal delivery," I replied.

"The day will come when you will understand the *gestalt of medicine,"* he replied. "It will take about ten years after your residency."

This made no sense to me. Bill sounded like Obi-Wan Kenobi, the Jedi master of Star Wars—"May the force will be with you." About ten years later, I was attending rounds with the residents at our inner-city hospital. We had finished seeing all of the patients on in the Labor unit and were completing rounds in the recovery room— an open ward where all the patients were watched for several hours after their C-sections before they were transferred to the postpartum floor. The residents presented a patient to me in the first bed: Twenty-five-year-old G3P2Ab1 (three pregnancies—two had resulted in babies and one had ended in miscarriage). She has just undergone a C-section for severe pre-eclampsia.

"We are watching her blood pressure which is a bit elevated so we have given her magnesium sulfate to prevent seizures," said the supervising resident.

I asked the patient how she was doing. "I dunno, Doc, but I got this really bad pain under the ribs on my right side," she replied.

I turned to the eight residents behind me, "I'm worried about a ruptured liver." Turning back toward the patient, I asked her, "Mind if I press on you a little over there?" I pressed deeply into the patient's right upper abdomen and she winced in pain.

"Can I get an ultrasound machine here?" I asked the residents. A small portable machine was wheeled over to the bedside. I squeezed a bottle of cold gel on the patient's abdomen.

"Sorry about that. They don't keep gel bottle warmers here at this hospital," I said.

When the machine finally warmed up and the image appeared on the screen, I could make out a rim of dark-appearing fluid under the patient's ribs and behind the liver—blood.

"A ruptured liver hematoma, guys. We need to take her back and evacuate this thing and pack her," I declared.

Moments later our patient was back in the operating room asleep with a breathing tube in her throat courtesy of our anesthesiologist. We opened her abdomen to find several pints of blood present. We removed the clots over her liver, placed large packs and drains, and closed things up. She would survive to have another child. The force was now with me!

I have given Bill's *gestalt of medicine* a lot of thought through the years. I have come to realize that the reason I knew that this particular patient had a liver hematoma was that I had already taken care of nine other patients with the same diagnosis during the course of my training. The majority had similar risk factors and symptoms. So, when my brain heard about and saw this patient, the clinical pattern was similar to the one that I had seen several times earlier. My brain had *muscle memory* , just like Venus Williams. In this case it was not a physical task that I had mastered. Instead, it was the ability to assimilate a series of facts into the most likely diagnosis. This only comes with experience. In my case, I happened to be at an institution where over the previous decade the denominator of pregnant women who might have this particular complication was 180,000. This resulted in my seeing nine previous cases of a rare condition.

10

Final Training—MFM Fellowship

Fellowship was the next step in my career. During OB-GYN residency training, a physician gains basic clinical skills and knowledge in the care of women. Fellowships allow for further refinement of new subspecialty skills. In the case of *MFM*, this includes the care of pregnant patients with medical complications. It also allowed the acquisition of skills in the emerging field of fetal medicine—ultrasound and fetal therapy. At that time, an MFM fellowship was a two-year training period, with time specifically allotted to research. Although residency does not allow any commitment to research time, MFM fellows are required to complete a prospective research project with subsequent publication in a peer-reviewed medical journal. Prospective research is not easy. One must develop an idea, get approval from a local ethics committee (called a *human investigational review board*), and then collect the data as the patients are enrolled in the study. This is followed by a statistical analysis of the results and then the need to write and submit the manuscript to a medical journal—no small task in a two-year period (today MFM fellows have three years to complete their thesis). Once the manuscript is submitted, the editor of the journal sends it out to experts in the field for *peer-review*. The best news is when the author receives a letter from the journal stating *accepted with major revision*. Changes are made based on the suggestions of the reviewers and the manuscript is resubmitted. The final anticipated letter is *accepted*. Actual publication in the journal may not occur until six months later. In today's age of the internet, the paper may appear in *PubMed* (the search engine for medical journals from the U.S. National Library of Medicine of the National Institutes of Health) as *Epub* (electronic publication) with a date indicating it has been accepted and is available online but is not yet in print.

At the start of the MFM fellowship, I really did not know what my future would hold. I had never been involved in biomedical research. And then there would be new clinical skills to learn. I soon realized that the presence of role models in medicine clearly influences one's path. Although I once thought that an individual should only have one mentor, it soon became apparent to me that one picks mentors based on their assets. The truth be known, few individuals in medicine represent the *triple threat*–clinician, teacher, and researcher. One learns to identify more than one mentor, each with their own set of skills.

Dr. Bill Wood was my clinical mentor. One day I was performing ultrasound with him in his office. He had just completed an uneventful *amniocentesis* (a procedure where a needle is placed into the amniotic fluid sac that surrounds the fetus) to check to see if the baby's lungs were ready for birth. That way an elective C-section delivery could be scheduled in this patient's second pregnancy. The patient's first pregnancy had been complicated by the birth of a little girl with *cloacal syndrome*—a congenital birth defect where the feces and urine empty into a common pouch instead of through the normal two separate openings. Even though this is not a lethal anomaly, the condition requires multiple surgeries early in a child's life to correct the problems. Wood was completing the ultrasound report on the patient. This allowed me the opportunity to pick up the transducer and do some ultrasound scanning myself. As I began to look at the baby's heart, I immediately realized something was wrong. The heart was barely beating. Maybe sixty times a minute (normal is 120 times per minute).

"Bill, can you take a look at this?" I said. Wood stood up, didn't say a word, and whisked out of the door. At this point the patient became suspicious.

"What's wrong?" she asked.

"Well, the heartbeat is a little slow and we are going to watch it here for a minute," I replied.

In what seemed like an eternity, the silence was interrupted by Dr. Wood bursting through the door of the room with a wheelchair.

"Let's go, get in," he instructed the patient. Down the hall we ran to the elevators. As luck would have it, Wood's office was on the sixth floor of the hospital and Labor and Delivery was just three floors below. We raced down the two-hundred-foot hall arriving at the elevators.

The elevator doors were closed and the elevator was on another floor.

"Damn, I locked it open. Someone must have unlocked it," he said. "Down the stairs we go."

Bill led the charge with the patient in the middle and me bringing up the rear. As we arrived in Labor and Delivery, we declared "stat C-section." Much to my dismay, our patient began to disrobe as she ran to the operating room. She had obviously been on Labor and Delivery before. By the time she jumped up onto the operating room table, she was completely nude.

"Put me to sleep now!" she told the anesthesiologist. We delivered the baby by emergency C-section within five minutes. The baby's Apgar scores were one and eight at one and five minutes of life. The little girl suffered bleeding into her lungs but ultimately made a complete recovery. She was discharged home a week later. We carefully examined the placenta and the umbilical cord—no signs of trauma. We never figured out what caused the fetal distress.

During fellowship, we were treated as junior attending physicians and were assigned our own patients who were transported to our *tertiary care* hospital from smaller outside institutions. A *tertiary care* hospital was usually one where any complication of pregnancy could be handled due to the presence of all the other major medical and surgical subspecialties. Today, the highest level of maternity care is designated by the American College of Obstetricians and Gynecologists as a *Level IV* hospital[23].

On this occasion, the patient arrived 28 weeks pregnant with twins. Her pregnancy was complicated by *pre-eclampsia* (high blood pressure) and *polyhydramnios* (too much amniotic fluid) in one of the twin's sac. I admitted her to our Labor and Delivery unit and checked out with one of the senior OB faculty to cover for the night. Later, the patient began to experience increasing abdominal pain in the upper right side of her abdomen. The obstetrical nurses called the attending and he advised treatment with morphine with the explanation that the extra amniotic fluid must be the source of her pain.

The next morning, I arrived for rounds. I took one look at my patient and I knew something was wrong. She was ashen and was writhing in pain.

"We are going to get you delivered by C-section," I informed her. "I am worried that your pre-eclampsia is getting worse." I then went to the doctor's lounge to change into surgical scrubs.

My patient's nurse stuck her head in, "Did you see her labs from this morning?" she asked. "Her platelet count is 20,000 (normal is about 150,000)."

"Wow, let's get her cross-matched for platelets and some red blood cells," I responded. I entered the operating room where the nurses had already painted the patient's abdomen with a brown anti-septic solution. The scrub tech had the sterile surgical drapes in place.

"Let's go ahead and put her to sleep," I instructed the anesthesiologist. I made a *Pfannenstiel* skin incision (a "bikini cut") and then entered the various tissue layers. As I cut into the last layer, bright red blood poured from the patient's abdomen.

She must have ruptured her uterus, I thought to myself.

I quickly felt around the womb—no tears but copious amounts of blood coming out from around it. I decided to get the twins delivered. I made a transverse incision in the uterus and easily delivered both baby boys. We handed them to the neonatologists and they were taken away to the neonatal intensive care unit. I quickly placed a large gauze pad in the uterus to stop the bleeding. Realizing that nothing was bleeding from the lower abdomen, I decided to make a second *vertical* (up and down) incision in the upper abdomen.

As I opened the various layers, I soon found the problem. There in the patient's right upper abdomen was the patient's liver covered by a large blood clot—a *hepatic hematoma*. This was a known complication of severe pre-eclampsia but I had only seen pictures of it in textbooks.

"Can you call Bill to come down from his office?" I requested of the circulating nurse. "I need to know what surgeon to call to help me."

Wood came running into the OR. "Cross-match her for ten units of platelets and six units of red cells!" he shouted.

"Bill, Bill, we're good," I said calmly. "We are already transfusing the patient. Who do I call for help?"

Dr. Peters, a general surgeon, showed up about twenty minutes later. He looked over the operative table.

"Never seen one of these before. Let me give my senior partner a call," he said.

He returned a few minutes later and scrubbed into the case. We removed the clot on the liver, placed large gauze packs on the oozing surface, and added large drains above and below the liver to remove any blood that might continue to accumulate. We then used surgical instruments to temporarily hold the patient's abdomen together. That night I kept transfusing blood into the patient. Finally, the blood count in the drain fluid became less than the blood count in her veins. I knew we had won the battle.

Two days later, we took the patient back to surgery and removed all of the gauze pads. No bleeding. After a stormy post-operative course, the patient was finally discharged home a month later. Her boys came home from the *neonatal intensive care unit* (NICU) two weeks later. This patient would be the first of more than a dozen patients I eventually experienced in my career with pregnancies complicated by pre-eclampsia with *liver hematomas*. These would all be challenging.

A few weeks after Rachael was born, I was supervising the OB-GYN residents at our inner-city hospital when I was called back to the OR. They had just completed the C-section on a patient with severe pre-eclampsia and her abdomen was full of blood. I suspected another liver hematoma.

"Go ahead and open up the top of her abdomen with a vertical incision and I will scrub in," I instructed. Three minutes later, after I had scrubbed and put on my gown and gloves, I peered into the incision.

"Just as I suspected a liver hematoma," I said. "Let's call general surgery over to give us a hand." Our hospital was located on the other end of town from the general hospital. For that reason, the general surgeons were all located at the trauma hospital, not at our obstetrical hospital.

I broke scrub and called the operator at the general hospital. "Can I speak the general surgery attending on call?" I asked.

"Let me put you on hold while I page them," she responded.

A few short minutes later, the surgeon answered. "Dr. Salvo here, whatcha got?" he questioned.

"I'm the MFM fellow on call here at the obstetrical hospital. We have a liver hematoma in a pregnant patient that we just sectioned and we need a hand," I said.

"Well just close her up and send her over to us by ambulance," he replied.

I returned to the OR to announce these instructions to the surgical team.

The attending anesthesiologist looked up from the head of the table. "You tell him this patient is not stable enough for transport and he needs to get his butt over here," she instructed.

I went back to the page operator, waited a few more moments, and was then speaking with Dr. Salvo again.

"Listen, the attending anesthesiologist really thinks the patient is not stable enough for transfer. She really wants you to come over," I explained.

"Dammit, Ok. I'll ride over in an ambulance," he responded.

Twenty minutes went by before Dr. Salvo appeared at the operating room door. He was clearly perturbed.

"How's her blood pressure doing?" he asked.

"Stable, but she has received three units of blood," came the reply from the anesthesiologist.

"Ok, I'll scrub in," said Salvo.

A few minutes later, he leaned over the open incision in the patient's abdomen. He reached over the liver and grabbed the large clot that was adherent to the top portion. Removing it was ease, he then threw it against the OR wall.

"Ok, towel clip her shut and transport her by ambulance to our hospital," he instructed. Then he turned and left.

We all looked at one another in dismay.

Based on my first patient with a liver hematoma, I decided to take charge. "Ok, we are going to need some large suction drains," I said.

The circulating nurse responded, "All we have are these small flat Jackson-Pratt drains in our hospital.

"These won't do," I answered. "Too small." I thought for a moment. "We are going to have to improvise. Open the crash cart and give me two *chest tubes*."

Chest tubes are large plastic drains that are placed through the chest wall to remove air or blood from around the lung usually after a car accident or other traumatic event. They could work well enough in our situation but I was concerned that the holes were so big that suction could cause the patient's bowel to become entrapped.

"Let me have some latex drains, as well," I said. "I'm going to sew these over the chest tubes and cut some small holes in them to keep the bowel from getting sucked in," I said.

We placed large packs over the oozing surface of the liver where Salvo had removed the hematoma. We then added our improvised drains above and below the liver and brought them out of the right side of the patient. Surgical *towel clips* (a clamp with teeth on each end) were used to hold her incision together. We then moved her to a stretcher and transported her by ambulance to the trauma hospital.

Sometimes medicine has strange rules that make little sense. I went to see the patient the next day at the trauma hospital. Our city has very hot summers and the standard dress for all physicians in our medical center was surgical scrubs and a white coat. In fact, physicians can even be seen at restaurants in our city wearing scrubs. As I was visiting the patient in the ICU, a surgical attending physician came up to me.

"You must leave this unit now," he demanded. "You are in the wrong color scrubs."

At the time I did not know who this individual was.

He shouted at me, "Do you know who I am?"

"Not really," I responded.

"I am Dr. Matthew, the attending physician who runs this ICU. You cannot be here in scrubs. Leave immediately."

"Interesting," I responded showing him my faculty badge. "I am an attending OB-GYN."

I decided it was not worth any more confrontation since I had already checked on my patient. I turned and walked away. Matthew followed me to the front door of the hospital.

The next day I learned that he had called my Chairman of OB-GYN to have me fired over the scrub incident. Despite this effort, I remained dutifully employed. I later found out Dr. Matthew was the chief of surgery at the general inner-city hospital. He was adamant that scrubs used in the surgical suite not be worn elsewhere in the hospital. This was to potentially prevent infection in surgical cases.

The actual data on surgical attire and its association with infection has only demonstrated that covering fascial and head hair with a cap and mask has any influence on the rate of surgical infection. Many hospitals however require that only scrubs of a special color be worn in operating rooms. Unfortunately, hospitals have been unable to make this practice convenient for physicians. Some have placed scrub vending machines in the physician lounge. These are often empty or the proper-sized scrubs are not available. Other hospitals issue a limited number of scrub sets to each physician. These are often laundered at home and worn into the hospital especially by residents in training.

Outside of infection and the practical issues, a patient's impression of physician attire has been the subject of several studies. Most of these have compared formal attire (collared shirt/tie/slacks or blouse/skirt) with white coat to a combination of surgical scrubs with a white coat[24]. Older patients preferred formal attire for physicians. However, in the majority of studies patients reported that the physician's attire did not affect their confidence in the physician. The combination of a white coat with scrubs was most acceptable in the emergency room or surgical area of the hospital. Clearly, the public's perception of a competent physician may be influenced by their images of the actors in their role as physicians on television shows.

Our hematoma patient was taken back to surgery the following day. This time I changed into the correct colored scrubs before entering the OR. I wanted to grab a few pictures of this rare complication of pregnancy. Anesthesia put the patient to sleep and the general surgery team removed the towel clips. They then took out the gauze pads we had left on top of the liver. Finally, they removed our two improvised drains.

The surgical chief resident looked at the drains. "What the heck are these?" he asked. "A chest tube with a latex drain sewn over it."

No one realized my identity in the back of the OR. I moved forward.

"Yep that's all we had at our little OB hospital. We made the best of it," I said.

"Looks like it worked," he replied.

Years later Dr. Matthew and I became friends when I was promoted to head of the obstetrical service at the same hospital where he remained as chief of surgery. In that role, I purchased my own monogramed scrubs for daily use. I made sure their color did not match those worn in his operating rooms.

About five years after we first met, I was leaving the hospital when I noticed Dr. Matthew headed my way. I put down my briefcase in dismay.

"I see you are wearing scrubs into the hospital," I said as I greeted him. He grinned back at me.

11

Bitten by the Research Bug

Expanding my clinical knowledge in complicated pregnancies was a key aspect of the fellowship. I was naïve to the other major component of my training—research. One of my mentors advised me to develop an area of medical research where no one else was doing much investigation.

"Do all the studies you can in that particular area," he said. "Develop a niche. Publish papers in major medical journals. Become known as the expert. Then they will ask you to write the chapters in the major textbooks and give lectures on that topic." This was good advice which I took to heart.

I would have to develop a research thesis as required to be able to be certified as an MFM specialist. In residency I had developed a curious interest in a particular drug that was said to be very effective for treating premature labor—*indomethacin. Premature delivery* (delivery of a pregnancy before 37 of 40 weeks) complicates almost 10% of pregnancies. Although the etiology is multifactorial, many cases have no identifiable cause. In these cases, MFMs will recommend *tocolytics* (drugs to stop the contractions) and *steroids* (to help the unborn baby to accelerate its lung function so that it will not need as much oxygen support in the nursery). Many of these pregnancies result in premature babies that are admitted to *NICU* for long periods of time. The average daily costs are about $3500, with the total cost ranging from $50,000 to over a million dollars[25]. The average length of stay in the ICU for all premature babies is about three weeks; however, *micro-premies* (those born between 24 and 28 weeks of pregnancy) will have very prolonged stays in the hospital. Efforts to prevent prematurity in our country have been disappointing, although survival of these babies has markedly improved with advancements in neonatal care.

Indomethacin is like a super aspirin. This non-steroidal drug blocks the production of a family of chemicals produced in our bodies during inflammation—*prostaglandins*. Certain *prostaglandins* are released at the time of premature labor, making the pregnant uterus contract. *Indomethacin* will quiet the uterus within just a few hours of taking the first oral dose. But *indomethacin* can cross the placenta to the fetus and stop the production of prostaglandins there as well. Animal studies had shown that the drug could cause a special blood vessel in the fetal heart to constrict—the *ductus arteriosus* (*ductus* for short)[26]. This small vessel normally closes a few days after a baby is born. But when the baby is still in its mother's womb, it acts like a bypass circuit, allowing blood from the right side of the heart to be directed away from the baby's lungs that are collapsed since the baby is not breathing air yet. If this vessel is affected while the baby is still in the womb, blood will be diverted to the collapsed lungs, causing damage to them. These concerns led MFMs to be wary of the use indomethacin for the treatment of premature labor.

I first poured over the medical literature. Today one can access the internet, log on to the *PubMed* site or *Google Scholar*, and search the world's medical literature with a few clicks of a mouse. Through our university medical library, one can then download a pdf file of the article, print the file, and presto—the info is there in two minutes. It wasn't that easy when I was a fellow. I had to go to our medical library and comb through years of *Index Medicus* bound volumes. I would then make a list of articles I wanted. Finally, I would drag a wooden carousel on wheels around the library to the rows of shelved hard-bound medical journals. After I found the correct volume, I would mark the pages of the article with a small slip of paper and then add the volume onto the carousel. Next was a trip to the copy machine and adding ten cents in change to copy each page of the papers I had selected. The redeeming factor of the library was that they insisted on re-shelving the hard volumes of the journals to ensure their proper placement for the next researcher.

I decided that *indomethacin* could affect the *ductus* but this did not appear to happen as much when the human fetus was premature—a time when we would want to use the drug to treat premature contractions. It was my good fortune to meet the next significant mentor in my early academic career. Dr. Hughes was one of those eccentric but brilliant physicians who had a passion for research. He was a *pediatric cardiologist* who has a special interest in doing fetal heart ultrasound (*fetal echocardiography*). What better person to help me with my research? As luck would have it, Dr. Hughes had some funds to do a sheep study on the ductus.

"Ever done any sheep research?" he asked me at our first meeting. "Want to take this project on?"

"You bet," I responded. "When do we start?"

A few weeks later I found myself in a small operating room on the second floor of the medical school facing a very large pregnant sheep lying on her side. She had been put to sleep by the veterinary technician and had a breathing tube in her throat.

"This is a non-survival surgery so you don't have to do things in a sterile fashion," she remarked.

As a trained obstetrician, it was easy enough to start the procedure and open the uterus to expose the fetus. I delivered the lamb to the level of the chest but left it connected to the umbilical cord. Then I was in new territory. I opened the chest and dissected down to the beating heart. I followed the *pulmonary artery* to what I thought was the *ductus*. While trying to place a clamp under the vessel, it ruptured and the fetus bled to death in front of my eyes (thank God it was asleep).

I called Dr. Hughes. "I think I need someone to come over and give me a hand on the next sheep if this is going to work," I said.

He made arrangements to have a senior pediatric cardiologist attend the next case. Things went much better. We grasped the front limb of the fetus this time and made a small incision on the side of the chest. This made for easy access to the *ductus*. We are able to place a small rubber tube around the vessel so that we could open and close it. Dr. Hughes came over and we did multiple ultrasound measurements opening and closing the ductus with the rubber tube.

Dr. Hughes was excited, "See there, when you close the vessel down, the measurement of the blood moving through it changes dramatically on ultrasound. Just as I predicted. This is fantastic!"

The next experiment did not go so well. Dr. Hughes sent over a visiting Israeli physician in training to assist me with the surgery. The first step of the procedure was to place an IV in the leg of the pregnant ewe once it was asleep. We also had to shear the wool from the abdomen to allow us to do the surgery. A small bottle of alcohol was used to spray the oily wool to allow the electronic clipper to cut more efficiently. I was placing the IV using the *electric cautery* (a pen-like device that uses electrical current to cut and coagulate bleeding vessels). As I was doing my procedure, my Israeli friend managed to spray alcohol onto my surgical site. I glanced up to see my entire pregnant sheep under a blue flame. It was on fire! I removed my surgical cap and tried to put out the flames but my cap caught fire too. My partner in crime handed me the fire extinguisher from the wall. He had no idea how to use it. I pulled the pin and with one blast of CO2, the flames were out. The sheep was still be ventilated and it appeared unaffected.

"She still has good vital signs," I said. "And no wool, let's move forward with the surgery?"

As we entered the abdomen, something was wrong. The uterus was filled with multiple fibroids and there were *adhesions* (scar tissue) everywhere. When we were finally able to open the uterus, we found that the fetus was dead—by the discoloration and size, it had been dead for several weeks. I later learned I was in violation of a medical school rule. I had not completed the fire report for the experiment!

Six sheep experiments later, Dr. Hughes declared we had enough measurements for a manuscript. He wrote the paper with me as the second author—a satisfying start to an academic career![27]

Now that we had established a way to detect decreased flow in the ductus, the next step was to design a human study. With input from several faculty, I submitted a protocol to the *human institutional review board (IRB)*. We picked patients in premature labor that needed treatment. A special ultrasound (*fetal echocardiogram*) would be performed before starting treatment and then we would look at the baby's heart several times over a forty-eight-hour period to make sure there were no ill effects of the indomethacin. The fellowship program did not have any funding to cover the expenses for the research, so I would have to negotiate all the testing. Dr. Hughes was willing to come in to do all the fetal echocardiograms with me at no cost. We decided to check the blood level of indomethacin in the mothers to see if this predicted any effects in the fetus. For this, I found a PhD at the Children's Hospital who was willing to run these at no cost in return for authorship on a manuscript. The IRB approved the study.

I still have a vivid memory of the first patient that I was to enroll in my first clinical research project. She was a young woman with her second baby at 26 weeks gestation who had been admitted to our inner-city hospital with premature contractions. We did the baseline echo and everything looked fine, so we started the indomethacin. By four hours later, her contractions had stopped and it was time for the first echo study on the drug. Much to my dismay, the baby showed evidence of severe constriction of the ductus. I was devastated! I just knew we had done something bad to this baby. We stopped the drug and switched to another one to keep the contractions stopped. I did not sleep that night. What had we done? My thesis project was over! Dr. Hughes assured me everything would be fine. But how did he know this?

The next day we repeated the echo, and the ductus had reopened. Thank God! I called the IRB and reported the problem. They wanted me to wait until the baby was born to be sure it was OK. Three months went by—what seemed like an eternity. The baby was born and his heart looked good. The IRB let me resume the study. We enrolled a total of fourteen patients in the study and half of them demonstrated some constriction of the ductus. The vessel always reopened after we stopped the drug. This had never before been reported in the human fetus. I made all the faculty swear to silence— no talking about the study at national meetings when having drinks at the bar with colleagues. I decided to submit the work to the *New England Journal of Medicine*—one of the most prestigious of medical journals having been first published in 1812. Several of my faculty discouraged me from submitting to this journal. After all I was an obstetrician from a southwestern state, not from a medical school in the New England area. I submitted it anyway. Several weeks later the letter arrived. I opened the envelop with hesitation—surely the article would be rejected. Instead, the first line read "We are pleased to inform you that your article is accepted with revision." I made the changes and sent it back to the journal within a week. The draft returned after undergoing significant editing by the English majors at the journal. Was this still my article? It had been changed so much. In any event, we finally were able to come to terms on the final version of the manuscript and I was the proud author of a *New England Journal of Medicine* publication[28].

Sometimes politics gets in the way of research.

"When you have lemons, make lemonade," a mentor once told me.

This was another piece of great advice regarding clinical research. In other words, don't decide to study some obscure disease if there aren't that many patients around in your medical center. Study the diseases that are more prevalent. I would later pass this advice on to the many junior faculty that I would mentor later in my academic career.

Indomethacin seemed to be my "niche." We knew virtually nothing on how the drug crossed the placenta during the pregnancy. Perhaps it did not cross over to the fetus in the early part of pregnancy, so it would be safer to use it then for the treatment of premature labor. At the time, Dr. Wood and I were very busy on the clinical service, taking care of patients with Rh disease. There had been significant progress in the technical aspects of the intrauterine procedure that was used to treat anemia in these fetuses. Unlike the procedure I had seen Bogs perform at the end of my residency, fetal transfusions were now performed with ultrasound, thereby eliminating the exposure of the developing fetus to repeated X-rays[29]. More importantly, based on some work done by an investigator in France, it was now possible to actually pierce the umbilical cord of the fetus to take a sample of blood to directly measure the blood count[30]. One could then infuse red blood cells with the same needle to correct the anemia. The *intravascular intrauterine transfusion method* began to save severely anemic fetuses that the older method of *intraperitoneal transfusion* could not save. But I thought, what an opportunity to study blood levels of indomethacin in these fetuses since they were requiring the umbilical cord puncture anyway. In addition, any small blood sample that we would need for the study would be easily replaced with the transfused red blood cells we were giving to correct the fetal anemia. In addition, patients often experienced contractions after the intrauterine transfusion procedure, so administering one dose of indomethacin to them before the procedure made good medical sense. The IRB agreed with my premises and the study was approved. Since patients undergoing intrauterine transfusion typically undergo four to six procedures for the treatment of the fetal anemia as they progress in pregnancy, we were able to acquire paired maternal and fetal samples on multiple occasions even in the same fetus. After collecting a sufficient number of samples (and promising authorship to my PhD colleague in the lab to run all the samples), the manuscript was submitted to the prestigious *American Journal of Obstetrics and Gynecology* journal.

Nifedipine, a new drug at the time for the treatment of high blood pressure, was also known to relax the muscles of the uterus much like it relaxes the smooth muscle of one's arteries. Studies in sheep had suggested however that acid might build up in the fetus if a similar drug was given to treat premature labor[31]. Dr. Bale, one of the other attending MFMs in our Division, knew of my indomethacin study and decided to use the technique of *cordocentesis* (ultrasound is used to guide a needle into the vein in the umbilical cord of the fetus) to measure the acid level in patients given nifedipine for premature labor. Only in this case there was no clinical rationale for the mother, and more importantly the fetus, to incur the risks of the procedure. These risks were not inconsequential and included fetal *bradycardia* (an extreme slowing of the fetal heart rate with the need for emergency delivery by C-section) and even fetal death. Dr. Bale asked me to be a co-investigator on the submission to the IRB. I refused for ethical reasons. Much to my dismay, the IRB did however approve his study. The second patient enrolled in the study was a young woman at 28 weeks gestation in premature labor. The cordocentesis was performed by a first-year MFM fellow with little experience with the procedure. A fetal bradycardia ensued and the patient was delivered by emergency C-section. The child was admitted to the NICU and after a prolonged neonatal course was discharged in good condition. Much to my surprise, once the IRB was notified of the complication, they allowed the study to continue. The data was eventually submitted to the same medical journal that was reviewing my indomethacin study.

The reviewers of Dr. Bale's paper decided it was entirely unethical to have undertaken the study and, despite IRB approval, sent a letter of sanction to all the authors on the paper. Dr. Bale responded to the journal that he was simply following the same protocol I was—both studies involved the study of how a drug crossed the placenta and both involved the same risks to the fetus. I soon received a similar sanction letter from the journal stating that "we do not know what the clinical investigators are doing at your institution but there appears to be a pattern of disregard for the fetal risks of this research." I immediately called the editor of the journal to explain the difference—my protocol involved fetuses who had a clinical indication for the umbilical cord puncture. Dr. Bale's study involved an elective procedure done only for the purpose of the study.

"Now I understand," replied the editor. "Big difference." A letter of acceptance for my study arrived from the journal three days later[32]. Dr. Bale's study was never published.

Research on human subjects has been plagued with tales of unethical experimentation. In 1941, German physicians at the Dachau concentration camp performed experiments on Jewish prisoners to determine the effects of cold-water emersion[33]. In the initial series of experiments, subjects were placed into freezing water of different temperatures to see how long their bodies could endure hypothermia before death ensued. Later experiments involved "rewarming" methods to see if recovery could be achieved. The rationale for these studies was to enhance the survival of German sailors that might have to abandon their sinking ships in freezing waters during World War II. More infamous was the Tuskegee Syphilis Study that took place in Alabama between 1932 and 1972[34]. More than 400 African American men with syphilis were provided "free medical care" by the U.S. Public Health Service. When penicillin became the *standard of care* for the cure of syphilis in 1947, therapy was withheld from these individuals to allow for the study of the natural progression of the disease. Many of the men went on to die from neurosyphilis—a late manifestation of progressive disease. In the interim, forty of their wives were infected and twenty-nine children were born with congenital syphilis. Once the U.S. government became aware of these experiments, the *National Research Act* was passed in 1974, establishing the *National Commission for the Protection of Human Subjects of Biomedical and Behavioral Research*[35]. Four years later, the *Belmont Report* outlined specific guidelines for the development of local *institutional review boards (IRBs)* to oversee the ethical treatment of patients participating in medical studies[36]. Paramount to these guidelines were the issues of informed consent and the providing of minimal medical care.

Today, all medical researchers must complete initial and ongoing education on the ethics of medical research. This is typically accomplished through web-based tutorials that are updated regularly. All medical schools and universities have IRBs where investigators must submit their research protocols. Studies cannot be initiated until approval is received. Patient enrollment and any complications are reported on an annual basis before the study is renewed. More recently, with the passage of the *Health Insurance Portability and Accountability Act (HIPPA)* in 1996, special attention is given to patient confidentiality in the collection of all personal identifiable data[37].

Yet medical researchers in other parts of the world have continued to push the envelope of ethics in medical research. Between 1973 and 1986, Dr. Green at the Auckland National Women's Hospital elected to follow over 100 women with *carcinoma in situ of the cervix* (a pre-cancerous lesion) to see how many patients would progress to invasive cancer[38]. The *standard of care* at the time was to offer these patients surgical removal of their pre-invasive lesions. In the early 2000s, Dr. Hwang at the Seoul National University was accused of coercing female technicians in his laboratory to donate their eggs for medical research[39].

I had learned a lot in my two years of MFM fellowship. One of our *off-service rotations* was a one-month assignment on the genetics service. During this time, we were assigned to see the patient first, then we would come back in the afternoon each day and present the patient to the attending faculty geneticist. The majority of the consultations were for women who had recently delivered an abnormal baby. At the end of the rotation, the head of the genetics fellowship pulled me aside.

"You have done a great job on the consults," he said. We would be very interested in your joining our genetics fellowship for the next two years after you have completed the MFM fellowship."

"I would be honored but let me talk with my wife first," I replied.

After all, at the time there were only a handful of faculty in the country who were double boarded in MFM and genetics.

I returned home that day to chat with my wife Karen.

"Say, they offered for me to start a genetics fellowship after I complete the MFM fellowship," I said.

Karen and I had married in my senior year of my residency. In our short marriage of two years, she had been my rock. She had applied to midwifery school and was accepted. Then we were blessed with an unplanned pregnancy. The midwifery training program required an out-of-state elective for several months and she could not see herself doing that with a new baby. So she decided to not to go to midwifery school. During the previous two years, she had basically been a single mom. Fellowship devoured my time and I was often sleeping after being on call the previous night.

"You are kidding, right," she replied. "Have you seen the credit card bills? It's time to get a real job." That made sense—I had been in training for six years and things were tight financially with Karen deciding to stop working as a nurse to stay home with Rachael.

At the end of fellowship, one must decide to enter private practice or to apply for a position as a faculty physician at a medical school, so called *academic medicine*. Private MFMs make significant impacts on their patients' lives. The true *triple threat* physician in academia demonstrates excellence in three areas—clinical care, research and teaching. These latter two areas allow the academic physician to move the field of medicine forward. Clinical research allows for new cures and better patient outcomes. Teaching passes knowledge on to the next generation of physicians who will care for many patients.

Later in my career, I was trying to recruit a physician who had been in private practice for many years to join our faculty at the medical school. I made the analogy of teaching to the proverbial pebble thrown into the pond. The ripples extend in ever-increasing circles that get larger and larger as they extend from where the stone first entered the pond.

"How many patients do you think you have cared for over the course of your career?" I asked.

"Perhaps a thousand," he responded.

"Think about this—if each year you train our twelve OB-GYN residents to take care of patients—they will each care for 1,000 patients in their lifetime. And you will influence a new class of twelve trainees every year," I said. Realizing the impact of my statement, he signed with the department the following day.

I graciously declined the genetic fellowship the next day. I would move on with the next phase of my life—Assistant Professor at a major medical school.

12

My First Real Job—
Assistant Professor

Our OB-GYN department had a unique financial system for faculty reimbursement. All faculty received a minimal base salary. Income from private patient care was used to supplement the salary to make it competitive with positions in private practice. One could keep 50% of collections once expenses were covered. These included a tax to the medical school, a departmental tax, malpractice premiums, and personnel salaries. My co-fellow and I negotiated our new faculty positions to include a full-time research nurse assigned to each of us. This is unheard of in today's job recruitment when most departments have little if any research infrastructure. I am convinced my first research nurse Lorrie was one of the main contributors to my early success in academic medicine.

East and I entered the department as Assistant Professors with a commitment to make teaching rounds at least one day each week at the inner-city obstetrical hospital where our residents received most of their OB experience. This meant that an attending would now formally round each day of the week—a radical change from the past where the senior residents ran the show by themselves with almost no faculty supervision.

Given our family financial situation, I started in my Assistant Professor position the day after I completed by MFM fellowship. I went into practice with Dr. Wood. The agreement was that we would cover our own patients on most weeknights and cross-cover every other weekend. For reasons that escape me, I remember not coming home for three straight nights in that first week in July.

I thought to myself, "I am an attending now, shouldn't things get easier?"

I was cross-covering Bill's practice one weekend when I received an unusual phone call from the answering service on Friday night. The mother of one of his pregnant patients was calling.

"I am very concerned about my daughter. She is 30 weeks pregnant. I have never seen her this sick," she said. "She missed her OB clinic appointment today. But please do not tell her I am calling you. She will be upset with me."

"Well, I'm not sure I can do anything if she does not call in, but let me give this some thought," I replied.

A few minutes after the call, I came up with the idea that I should call the patient with the excuse that she had missed her prenatal appointment and I was simply following up to be sure everything was fine. Her husband answered the phone.

"This is Dr. Moise, one of Dr. Wood's associates, I understand that your wife missed her OB appointment today and I am calling to check in with her. Can she come to the phone?" I questioned.

"She's in bed not feeling very well, so I don't think she can come to the phone," he responded.

"So what's specifically going on with her?" I inquired.

"She hasn't eaten very much in the last few days and her temperature has been running a bit high—about 103 degrees," he replied.

"Maybe you should go ahead and bring her into Labor and Delivery so we can take a look at her," I instructed.

About an hour later the patient arrived. Most women are healthy when they are pregnant. After all most are young and have few medical problems. This was not the case with this patient. One look at her and I knew she was sick. Her initial temperature was 102 degrees. She had no real complaints other than "I don't feel good." I did a complete head to toe physical exam. I thought there might be some mild *nuchal rigidity* (neck stiffness)—a possible sign of *meningitis* (an infection of the layers of tissue surrounding the brain). There were no signs of tenderness over the uterus, a sign of possible infection around the fetus. Blood work indicated a very high white blood cell count, indicating there could be an infection somewhere. Her urinalysis was clean—no kidney infection. I was perplexed.

"I think we should do an amniocentesis to check for any infection in the womb. This would be unusual with your bag of waters being intact but I can't figure out where your fever is coming from," I said.

She and her husband agreed to the procedure. The procedure was easy. The fluid results came back an hour later—no signs of infection.

"I think I am going to ask one of our infectious disease consultants to look you over with me," I said.

An hour later my consultant arrived. I told him the story and suggested we consider a spinal tap for possible *meningitis*.

"Let me look her over a bit if you don't mind," he replied. As a young attending, I was always impressed with the physical exam skills of the senior physicians.

"Ken, did you see these splinter hemorrhages in her nails?" he asked.

I looked over his shoulder. How could I have missed these? A classic medical student sign of *bacterial endocarditis*. When there is an infection of the heart valves, small amounts of bacteria break off and move through the patient's bloodstream. They lodge in the small capillaries in the nail beds and present as small areas of bleeding. We decided to take several blood cultures, put the patient on powerful antibiotics, and get a special ultrasound of the patient's heart (*echo-cardiogram*). Sure enough, there it was—a big bacterial *vegetation* (growth) on the *aortic valve*, the valve that opens to the large blood vessel coming from the left side of the heart to supply blood to the rest of the body. A day later the blood cultures confirmed the infection—*Staphylococcus aureus*, a virulent bacteria known to infect heart valves.

"Glad you caught this," my consultant told me a few days later. "Left untreated she would probably have died in a week or so."

"Thank her mom," I said.

After a week of powerful antibiotics, the infection had still not cleared. The cardiovascular surgeon decided in consultation with infectious disease that replacement of the valve was the only recourse. So, Bill took his patient to C-section at 31 weeks. The patient was delivered in the cardiovascular surgery suite so that she could be placed on *cardiac bypass* right after the C-section (the patient is placed on a heart/lung machine to put oxygen in her blood while the heart is stopped for the surgery). The surgeon opened her chest and removed the diseased valve. Still showing signs of infection, it looked like Swiss cheese as he cut the valve away. He then replaced it with a metal valve. When the pathology on the valve returned, we had our answer as to why the patient developed this rare condition. She was born with a *bicuspid aortic valve*. Normally the *aortic valve* has three flaps that close. But in 1% of individuals, the valve only forms with two flaps. This results in the valve not closing normally putting the valve at risk for infection if any bacteria get into the patient's bloodstream. Arnold Schwarzenegger was probably the most famous person who had his bicuspid aortic valve replaced in 1997[40]. Bill's patient made a full recovery. Her infant girl was discharged from the NICU several months later.

Being an attending, can be very intimidating at first. When you are a resident or fellow, there is always the attending to consult for advice. When you are the attending, the buck stops with you. One of the patients referred to me in my practice was in her fourth pregnancy. This African-American woman was older than most of my patients being around forty years of age. She was clearly the matriarch of her family. Unfortunately, she had been diagnosed with a rare form of metastatic breast cancer. The cancer cells had actually entered the *lymphatic system* of her lungs.

Lymph nodes are the guardians of our bodies. Connected in a large network through a series of channels, they filter out cancer cells before they can metastasize around our body. The lymphatic channels in the lungs also remove extra water that accumulates from the air pockets. This was the concern for my patient. How would she handle the normal movement of fluids that would happen in her body after her baby was born? Throughout her pregnancy, we had multiple conversations regarding her decisions on life support if she became terminally ill.

"I do not want to be intubated on a ventilator," she said. "Anything else but that."

As her pregnancy progressed, her shortness of breath continued to get worse. We placed her on home oxygen therapy. Finally, at around 30 weeks gestation, a measure of the oxygen in blood indicated that it was low enough to put her unborn child at risk.

I explained to her, "I think we should get you delivered by C-section. We will put a breathing tube in for the surgery but we will take it out in the recovery room." She agreed.

She had to sit up due to shortness of breath for the anesthesiologist to place the breathing tube for the surgery. The MFM fellow and I did what was probably the quickest C-section I had ever done. From skin incision, to delivery, to skin closure probably took less than fifteen minutes. We managed to remove the breathing tube in the recovery room as I had promised. For the first few hours after delivery, providing oxygen by a plastic face mask was sufficient to maintain the oxygen level in my patient's bloodstream. But after about twelve hours, my earlier fears became a reality. No one is really quite sure why fluids begin to shift in the first few days after a baby is born. *Edema* (extra water in the tissues) in various parts of the body begins to mobilize into the bloodstream. Normally the kidneys can take care of this, but if there is too much fluid, then *pulmonary edema* (fluid in the air spaces of the lung) can occur. Normally the *lymphatics* can clear this fluid with the help of powerful diuretic drugs to stimulate the kidneys. But my patient's *lymphatics* were filled with cancer cells. Her oxygen levels declined progressively. Powerful diuretics did not seem to have any impact.

A *CPAP* mask (a way to provide oxygen under pressure without using a breathing tube) was the final step. Even this did not work. My patient's breathing became more and more labored. Finally, I decided to sedate her with morphine to ease her discomfort. She took one last deep breath a few minutes later and passed away peacefully.

Later that day, I was called by the nurses to meet with the family. I walked into the room where more than twenty family members waited for me. The anger in the room was palpable.

Her oldest son was the spokesperson for the group. "Why did you let our mother die?" he asked. "Why didn't you put in a breathing tube and put her on a ventilator?"

"Your mother and I had many conversations about what she wanted after the baby was delivered. We talked about what might happen and she told me she did not want heroic measures to prolong her life. I agreed with her plan given that she was not going to be able to live much longer with her breast cancer," I responded.

A daughter spoke up. "This baby caused her to die. Why didn't you just let the baby die inside her?" she asked.

"This was not what she wanted either," I replied.

The family left the meeting still angry over the loss of their mother. No one came to see the baby in the nursery for three weeks. Obviously, their anger was displaced on the baby as well. Arrangements were being made by the social worker to place the baby in foster care. The oldest daughter of my patient finally showed and took the child home to raise.

After practicing with Dr. Wood for one year, I decided I could not keep pace with this energetic physician who was ten years my senior. My co-fellow, East, also decided that a life caring almost exclusively for private patients as part of an appointment to the medical school was not his calling. He left the university to move north. I realized I had also been bitten by the academic bug. I wanted to spend more time teaching and doing research. This meant a major cut in salary, but I would be able to spend four days each week with the OB-GYN residents at the inner-city hospital. I would receive the additional base salary originally assigned to East. Each Friday I would see private patients to pay my other expenses.

I was once at a dinner party, when a young woman said to me. "So, I hear you teach at the medical school."

It has been my impression that the general public believes that professors at a medical school spend most of their time at the head of a classroom providing a lecture to their students. Professors of anatomy or biochemistry do provide this type of instruction in the basic science years of medical school. During the clinical years of training, we are occasionally called upon to give lectures using overhead projected slides in dark rooms. But the clinical teaching of medical students and residents occurs in the hospital. Some institutions do this in the form of a *morning report*—a meeting in a conference room near the patient care area. Medical students and residents assigned to the *service* meet with the supervising attending professor. Each patient's demographics are presented and a plan of care is formulated. On the obstetrical service, this meeting usually occurs at the *board*. Once centrally located in the middle of Labor and Delivery, new *HIPPA* rules of patient privacy have changed the location to a back room. Originally, the *board* consisted of a large white dry erase panel interlaced with black (brown) lines. Patient names, their gestational age, the number and outcomes of their previous pregnancies, and the status of their cervical dilation were prominently displayed. On the far right was a column for a plan of care. Today, computer screens have replaced the white board. Complete patient names are replaced by initials—a dehumanizing consequence of *HIPPA* regulations.

As an Assistant Professor, we do not receive instruction on how to teach patient care to our trainees. We learn by observation of the more senior professors and develop our own style of instruction. We all develop our own idiosyncrasies. Mine was that I immensely disliked the residents reading the facts on the labor board to me to present their patients. I preferred to make true *rounds. Rounds* is an interesting concept in medicine. The term is reported to be derived from the shape of the main inpatient building at the Johns Hopkins Hospital in Baltimore—the location of the first formal residency training program. It is rumored that Sir William Osler, the first professor at the newly formed Johns Hopkins School of Medicine in 1883, would walk from patient bed to bed with his residents to instruct them on the care of the patients. Since the original set of patient wards was in a round building, the residents soon coined the term *rounds*. During *rounds*, most professors teach using the *Socratic method.* A patient is presented and then a question is posed to the most junior trainee about some aspect of their care—usually the intern. If they cannot answer the question after a brief period, then the second-year resident is asked and so on. When no one can answer the question, one has the option of providing the answer or assigning an investigation to one of the residents so that they can provide the answer the next day on rounds. I felt it was important to make rounds at the bedside as Osler used to do. The patient and her family deserved to understand what we were thinking and planning for her care that day. Not all attendings agreed with this approach. My goal was to always have the students and residents leave rounds each day with at least one new piece of knowledge. *Rounds* were an opportunity to teach other concepts such as cost-effective health care as well. Often, I would quiz the residents on the costs of a medication or a test. They usually did not have any idea. I would make them research the costs and report at rounds the next day. I once heard of a professor who started his month on service by giving every resident $1,000 in Monopoly money. If during rounds he determined that an inappropriate test was ordered, the resident was assigned to investigate the cost and then pay the bank back in Monopoly money." "At the end of the month, I will give any resident that still has Monopoly money remaining the equivalent credit in books at the medical book store," he said. At the end of the rotation, all the residents owed the bank money. Another one of my idiosyncrasies was that I felt strongly that the entire team caring for the patient should attend rounds. Recent studies even in intensive care units have shown improved patient outcomes as a result of *team rounds*. On the obstetrical service, this mainly involved the individual OB nurse assigned to the patient and the *charge* (head) nurse for the unit for that shift. I married a nurse. She taught me the value of a team approach. Nurses can offer a different perspective to the patient's care.

I was rounding with our team on one occasion, when the resident presented a pregnant patient with infectious diarrhea. After the presentation was completed, the patient's nurse, standing in the rear of the circle of residents and medical students, interrupted, "You know she shares a common bathroom between the two labor rooms with the patient next door. Shouldn't we place her on some form of isolation precautions?"

"Great point," I said in admiration for a nurse who had the fortitude to speak up on rounds. This concept of including the nurses on rounds is also not embraced by all teaching attendings. They believe in a "us and them" separation between physicians and nurses. My wife tells me that in the first hospital where she worked, the OB nurses were required to follow the private attending into each patient's room carrying their charts and an ash tray (all doctors smoked in hospitals then!). Thankfully, there is now more mutual respect between physicians and nurses. Even today however, when a physician decides on a plan of care, he writes an *order* not a "request" for a medication to be given.

Of course, nursing has changed significantly in OB. Several decades earlier, the nurse was assigned to remain at the bedside to care for the patient in labor. This was especially true when the pregnant patient was being "induced"—an intravenous medication called Pitocin was used to stimulate uterine contractions. Nurses would place their hand on their patient's pregnant belly and feel for the tightening that occurs with the contractions. This would help time the contractions so that the Pitocin drip could be titrated to the proper rate. The nurse would also listen to the fetal heart rate after the contraction with a fetoscope—a special type of stethoscope. To increase the chance of hearing the baby's heartbeat, there was a plastic or metal bridge attached to the end of the stethoscope that the nurse placed onto her forehead and then pushed the device against her patient's pregnant belly. Drops in the heart beat were called decelerations. And then came the advent of electronic fetal monitoring. Two belts would be placed around the pregnant woman's belly. One would sense contractions and display them at the bottom of a continuous paper recording. A second belt could be adjusted to have an ultrasound sensor detect the unborn baby's heartbeat and display it on the top of the paper recording. This meant that the nurse was no longer required to remain at the bedside.

I was making bedside rounds in Labor and Delivery one day with a team of medical students and residents. We approached one of the laboring patients and I decided to challenge the observational skills of my team. "Tell me what is wrong with this patient," I asked.

The chief resident answered first. "Well the fetal heart rate monitor reveals a normal rate with no decelerations. The contractions are coming every three minutes. The patient has a *Foley* in place (a tube in her bladder to drain urine) and her urine appears to be clear. The intravenous fluids are running at 100 cc/hour (these were being administered by an electronic pump). There is an epidural pump working for pain relief. Everything looks OK to me."

"And where is the patient's nurse?" I asked. "The patient seems to be on autopilot!"

As a medical school professor, "teaching" expands past the boundaries of our local institution. As one gains expertise in certain clinical areas, we are asked to provide talks to national and international medical audiences. The art of presentation is another skill that one must acquire during the course of an academic career. There is no course on how to give a great presentation. My wife used to listen to some of my early talks to provide feedback.

"Tell them a patient story," she would say. "That will resonate with them much better than a bunch of words on a PowerPoint slide."

At one of my early presentations at a national meeting of OB-GYN's, an audience member came up to the podium at the end my talk. "Dr. Moise, you are the expert on this topic. Although I appreciate all the references to large studies, we came here for you to tell us how to manage our patients. Give us the "Cliff Notes" if you would."

This was a pivotal moment in my learning curve on giving presentations. From then on, my slides were limited to only a few bullet points. I would lean on the podium in a comfortable manner and tell the audience my experiences and how to care for their patients. I began to receive high evaluation scores for my talks.

The World Wide Web expands our teaching to even greater horizons. After a talk I gave in Peru, a local physician came up to greet me. "Can I get you to sign this textbook for me?" he said. "I read your chapter on Rh disease. I follow all of your publications on the topic. You have taught me how to care for my patients through your writings."

On one of the few afternoons when I had the time to ponder life, I decided that there are only three things that one leaves on this world once we depart—our children, our trainees, and the written word. To get all of these right, has been a driving force in my life.

I spent most of my time as an Assistant Professor at the inner-city hospital. With almost fifty pregnant women delivering a baby each day, medical students and family practice residents from other training programs did the majority of the normal deliveries. Residents did the forceps deliveries and C-sections. In fact, during the Christmas holiday, we would pay medical students who had completed their core OB rotation to work shifts to assist with normal deliveries. These "mercenaries" were paid from the "placental fund." In the basement of our hospital were several large freezers where we stored all the placentas from the 15,000 deliveries each year. The Avon company would come by annually to collect the placentas and pay the department one dollar per placenta. They were used as a source of human protein for cosmetics. Of course, HIV was not even on the horizon at that time.

Dr. Winkle was the Director of the MFM Division, the MFM fellowship and the Director of OB at this hospital. He had been at the institution for over twenty years. Until my arrival, *rounds* consisted of his daily appearance in the morning for about ten minutes. He would arrive in a dirty white coat with a cigarette in hand. His fingers were notably stained with nicotine from his many years of smoking.

"Any problems, boys?" was his classic line.

When told no, he would return to his office on the other side of the hospital never to be seen again that day. Dr. Winkle was at one time said to be a gifted surgeon, even training for one year as a surgical oncology fellow at a famed cancer institute in our town. But the many years had taken their toll and often he would arrive in the morning with an air of ethanol emanating on his breath. Knowing his shortcomings, he no longer participated in direct patient care but served mainly in an administrative position at the hospital.

Dr. Winkle had the wisdom of many years in obstetrics. I was once on the maternal transport service at the private hospital (where I still took call to pay expenses) when a referring physician called to ask what to do with his patient. She was 30 weeks pregnant and he claimed that her *cervix* (the opening to the womb) was prolapsing through her vagina down to the level of her knees. I did not believe this description. I had only seen pictures of this in textbooks. When the patient arrived by ambulance, I met her at the hospital. When I pulled back the sheets to examine her, I must admit I was stunned. Her uterus appeared to have descended through her vagina and now extended down to her mid thighs. "How long has this been like this?" I asked. "For about a week," she replied. "I was in bed this week until I saw my doctor for my regular OB visit this morning." Upon questioning, the patient related to me that she had been born with a birth defect that involved the formation of her vagina and rectum. She had undergone multiple surgeries as a child. Obviously, this birth defect had left her with a deficit in the normal support structures that keep the uterus in its normal position in the lower part of the body. In her case, the advancing size and weight of her pregnancy had allowed these deficiencies to become apparent. "You are a very unusual case," I told the patient. "Let me talk to some of my peers and get their opinion." I immediately called Dr. Winkle and told him what I was facing. "No problem. I've seen a couple of these," he said, not that I was surprised. "Just put her to sleep and *reduce* (push) the uterus back into the pelvis. Then put in a *doughnut pessary*. She will be fine." It took me awhile to find a doughnut pessary. Hospitals don't have them. TThey look like a rubber doughnut and are typically used in older patients who have some degree of uterine prolapse who do not want to go to surgery. The *pessary* is put in the upper part of the vagina and only removed every few months for cleaning. I asked one of the older OB-GYN's who happened to be waiting for one of his laboring patients to deliver that night, "Do you happen to have a doughnut pessary at your office?" "Sure," he replied. "What size do you need?"

"Not sure," I responded.

After his patient delivered, we headed to his nearby office and he pulled open an entire drawer of every form of vaginal pessary that exists. I picked a few different sizes of the type I needed and headed back to the hospital. Just as Dr. Winkle had suggested, I had the anesthesiologist put the patient to sleep and the uterus was easy to push back up into its proper position. I then placed the *pessary* in the upper part of the vagina—too easy. As the breathing tube was being removed from the patient's throat at the end of the procedure, she began to cough violently. *Oh, God*, I thought, *she is going to push it all out again*. I promptly grabbed a roll of surgical tape and taped her thighs together. Success! I sent the patient back to her OB-GYN a day later (after removing the tape). Several weeks later she presented to her referring hospital complaining of leaking amniotic fluid. Her doc called me again, "What should I do?" "Take out the *pessary* because we have to be concerned about infection," I responded. "But then she will prolapse again," he responded. "Yes, but then you can actually see if her cervix has dilated," I replied. He did find my comment amusing. The patient went on to have a successful vaginal delivery a few days later. Her uterus returned to its normal position after the she delivered.

Since I was spending the majority of my time at the inner-city hospital, I was eventually named as the Assistant Director of OB. We began to assess some long-standing practices that were being passed down resident to resident, with little change over time. Patients with medical complications of pregnancy like diabetes usually undergo special testing to see if their unborn baby is doing well. The *oxytocin challenge test (OCT)* was one of the original tests for fetal well-being. In this test, an IV is placed and the patient is given a drug to have enough uterine contractions to see if her fetus tolerates them. Basically, during a uterine contraction, the blood flow to the placenta stops and the fetus has to hold its breath. The normal fetus does fine with this. But if there are problems developing, the fetal heart rate drops during the contractions, signaling a potential problem. Although the test is a good one—it was falling into disfavor at many institutions. The patient had to be connected to an IV and once the uterine contractions were coming close enough and the fetus was looking OK, one turned off the medication. Then, the patient had to wait for several hours to be sure that she did not go into labor. On a busy Labor and Delivery unit, this meant about an eight-hour test. Canadian MFMs had introduced a new ultrasound test called a *biophysical profile (BPP)* which proved to be as good as the OCT.I trained a young OB-GYN from Mexico to do biophysical profiles.

Physicians born in other countries who then come to the U.S. make up almost one-fourth of our current workforce. We are one of the few countries that only accepts training in an American OB-GYN residency before a foreign-born physician can practice here. The one exception is Canadian-trained physicians who do not have to repeat their residency training. These foreign physicians are usually the brightest of the bright. In fact, the USA has often been accused of being the "brain drain" for developing countries since many of these physicians complete their residency and fellowship training and then do not return to their native country. All must pass all three parts of the national medical board examinations and an additional English proficiency exam. Only then can they compete with graduates of U.S. medical schools for residency training positions. Dr.

Lira aspired to get a residency position at our medical school in OB-GYN. Over the course of five years he performed several thousand BPPs. What was once an all-day test, was now completed in twenty minutes. Although the patients had to come to the hospital twice a week instead of only once a week when the OCT's were being used, they rarely complained. His exemplary work ethic led to Noe's eventual acceptance into our OB-GYN residency program. He is currently a very successful private OB-GYN in a southwestern state.

Magnesium sulfate is a salt that has been given since 1906 to prevent seizures in women with high blood pressure related to pregnancy (*eclampsia*). For many years it was given as an intramuscular shot. This was quite painful as it required an injection in each buttock, so the medication was often combined with a local anesthetic to help with the pain. In the mid-1980s, several U.S. hospitals began to give magnesium through an IV drip—a much more humane approach. This change was long overdue at our inner-city hospital. Patients were sent to the postpartum ward with orders for intramuscular magnesium every four hours. The nurses were told they could hold a dose if they determined that the patient was not urinating as much as expected. They could also hold the dose if they did not get a normal response when they attempted to elicit a *deep tendon reflex* (tapping on the knee joint to get the leg to jump forward). I began to notice that patients were being brought back down from the post-postpartum wards with seizures. *Eclampsia* still remains one of the major causes of maternal death in our country. Perhaps, the nurses were attempting to shield their patients from painful injections. More likely, there were simply not enough nurses on the postpartum ward with 18,000 pregnant patients delivering every year to give the magnesium every four hours. It was time for a change. We decided to retain all patients with *pre-eclampsia* (high blood pressure) in the Labor and Delivery recovery room immediately after delivery to receive intravenous magnesium. Six beds were set aside but it soon became apparent that we would fill these in the first few days. The standard protocol for intravenous magnesium administration at most academic hospitals at the time was to give the drug for twenty-four hours to all patients. This would not be possible due to our limited bed space. So, we implemented a policy that individualized the amount each patient would receive. The rule was a triple-digit urine production for three straight hours, then stop the magnesium. The rationale was that if the patient's kidneys were recovering from their disease, then so should their brains (*eclampsia* is thought to be the result of spasm of the small arteries in the brain). Our policy was implemented and much to our surprise the post-partum *eclamptic* seizures on the OB service became only a chance occurrence.

Our large obstetrical hospital was built in 1924, and after sixty-five years, it had outlived its usefulness. The Hospital District, a unique organization funded by city property taxes to care for the indigent patients, had decided to build two new hospitals. Although the contracts were signed to start construction of both at the same time, delays plagued the hospital located on the south side of the city so that its sister, north-located hospital, would be completed a year earlier. The original plan was for the north hospital to be for the care of low-risk pregnant women. It would be staffed by nurse midwives with some OB-GYN residents. The southern hospital would be for a smaller *high-risk* obstetrical population, since it was being constructed next to the other full-service inner-city hospital. Enter the world of politics. How could the taxpayers allow a brand-new hospital to sit unoccupied for one year while the southern hospital was being completed. And so we were told we would be moving our OB service to a building that was not constructed to handle 18,000 deliveries each year. Nevertheless, the day came when we closed the doors of our oldest institution. All delivered patients that could not be sent home were transferred by ambulance. Newly arriving patients in labor were directed to the new facility. Patients that had already been admitted in labor were allowed to deliver, then they were transferred to the new building with their babies in their arms. This meant of course organizing two teams of OB residents—one at each building for at least the first twenty-four hours. Needless to say, this was not well received by an already overworked group of young physicians. But everyone pitched in and the whole move came off without a hitch. We were adopting well to our new circumstance when politics struck again. The original low-risk/high-risk obstetrical patient plan for location of deliveries at the two new hospitals had been scrapped.

A significant change occurred in the responsibilities of our faculty during this year. The *AAMC* had ruled that a faculty member needed to be "immediately available" on a twenty-four-hour basis for coverage of our OB-GYN residents. This would mean that a faculty member would have to sleep in-house every night and on weekends at the inner-city hospital. No one liked this change. Often, the clinical professors would leave their assigned hospital in house call if one of their patients came into a nearby private hospital in labor. They seldom returned. Little was done to hold these individuals responsible for coverage. One Saturday evening, I was in my office studying for my OB-GYN board certification exam. I made several trips to the nurses' station to get water to make coffee so the resident staff knew I was on the premises. A few hours after my arrival, a second-year resident appeared at my office door with a look of fear in his eyes. "Dr. Short would like you to come out and see this patient he is having problems with."

"Where is the attending that is supposed to be in house?" I inquired.

"We have not seen him today. He called in earlier and said he would be at home if we needed him," he replied.

"Ok then, I'll have a look." When I arrived to the labor room where the resident directed me, there was no patient and no labor bed.

"Anyone know where this patient might me?" I asked the nursing staff.

"Dr. Short and the residents took her back for an emergency C-section," they answered. I quickly headed back to the operating room. When I opened the door, the scene was chaotic. The senior resident was on a stool performing chest compressions on a pregnant patient and the third-year resident was starting the C-section. I briefly washed my hands and put on a gown and gloves. When a pregnant patient has a cardiac arrest, removing the baby from the womb within four minutes accomplishes two things. The baby is more likely to survive without brain injury since maternal cardiac arrest will stop the flow of blood and oxygen to the uterus. More importantly, studies have shown that the mother has a greater chance for survival once the fetus has been delivered since the child is no longer using oxygen from the mother and chest compressions can be performed more effectively with the uterus now smaller in size after the delivery. So, we quickly performed the emergency C-section—the baby was out within five minutes. She survived with no hint of problems. Her mother was a not so lucky. After the fetus was out, the uterus refused to clamp down. Profuse bleeding began. We tried to close the incision in the womb that we had used to remove the baby, but the uterine muscle would not contract and the patient continued to lose blood. As a last-ditch effort, we started a hysterectomy to remove the bleeding uterus. But it was too late, the patient had not received enough oxygen to her brain and the pupils of her eyes remained fixed and dilated. She would not recover brain function. We decided to stop the code and the patient was declared dead.

Several months later, I received notification from an attorney. The patient's family intended to sue us for wrongful death. The claim was that we had missed an allergy to the penicillin that the residents had ordered to treat an infection that could have caused harm to the baby if it had been born through the birth canal. On later investigation, it was determined that the patient was not allergic to penicillin. The patient's autopsy revealed she had died from a rare condition called *amniotic fluid embolism*. I have only cared for five patients in my career with *amniotic fluid embolism*—they have all died. In this condition, amniotic fluid and fetal skin cells enter the pregnant woman's blood stream during labor. This causes a severe reaction that results in heart failure, a drop in blood pressure, and the inability of the blood to form clots to stop bleeding. The reason why this occurs is unknown. It is not predictable. The lawyers decided not to pursue the lawsuit when the results of the autopsy returned—this was an act of nature and not due to medical error.

The loss of a pregnant patient is devastating to the obstetrician and the OB nurses. In most cases, these women are young and healthy before calamity strikes. In my role as an attending physician at three major academic institutions, I have been involved in more than a dozen maternal deaths. These can rarely be predicted and often occur despite the best of medical care. A feeling of helplessness is accompanied by a significant burden of guilt. This is compounded by the fear of reprisal from the peer review process. All maternal deaths are labeled by hospitals as *sentinel events* and a *root cause analysis* is undertaken soon after the incident to see if the death had been preventable due to a medical error. This process only accentuates the guilt. Although healthcare workers play the primary role of providing support to the family in this difficult situation, we often do not take care of ourselves. At one of my positions as Chief of OB, I formed a maternal grief committee that was headed by an amazing non-denominational chaplain. All members of the healthcare team involved in the immediate care of the patient were invited to the meeting within twenty-four hours of the maternal death. I always attended these meetings. It was not uncommon to have tears flowing from physicians and nurses alike. They would often blame themselves for "missing something." Ultimately the staff were thankful for the experience because it allowed them to express their guilt and remorse for the loss of an otherwise healthy patient. I have not seen this committee duplicated at many other medical centers. Perhaps it is our reluctance to acknowledge that maternal death occurs. Perhaps it is our reluctance to understand that some events are beyond our control even with the best of medical care. In any event, we should take care of our own in these difficult times.

In 2019, it has been estimated that 810 women die daily in pregnancy or childbirth somewhere in the world—about one every 1.7 minutes of each day[41]. Most of these occur in the developing world. South Sudan has the worst rate of maternal mortality with 1,150 deaths per 100,000 births. By comparison, the USA ranks #60 in the world. The rate of 20.1 per 100,000 births in 2019 in our country is worse than any other developed country. A clear racial disparity is present, with African-American woman dying at a rate three times higher than their Caucasian counterparts. Today, the definition of maternal death proposed by the *World Health Organization* is a death from any cause from the start of pregnancy until forty-two days after delivery[42]. Late maternal deaths are defined as between forty-two days and one year after delivery. Maternal deaths are designated as *pregnancy-related* (like pre-eclampsia) or *non-pregnancy-related* (suicide and auto accidents). A further classification is *preventable* or *non-preventable*. Preventable deaths comprise about 60% of all maternal deaths. At present, the number-one cause of maternal death in the USA is drug overdose. Other causes include cardiovascular disease, bleeding, infection, and hypertensive disorders. Given our embarrassing international ranking, there are significant ongoing efforts to lower the rate of maternal mortality in the USA. Many states have formed maternal mortality review commissions to review data and assess trends that can be addressed. California has been especially successful in recent years in decreasing the rate of maternal mortality through state-wide efforts to standardize the treatment of hypertension and bleeding when the patient presents in labor.

After about a year in our new inner-city hospital, the sister hospital was finally completed and obstetrical services would be now need to be offered at both institutions. In the construction plans, my private medical school that had staffed the original inner-city hospital was to asked continue to provide obstetrical coverage for both new hospitals. Now the state medical school located in our city wanted in on the action. They would be assigned to the northern hospital and the private medical school would only provide services at the southern hospital. Patients would be told which hospital to use for their obstetrical delivery based on the zip code where they resided. There was only one fly in the ointment—the state medical school did not have enough OB-GYN residents to cover their new hospital. Solution—they approached the *American Board of OB-GYN* and were allowed to create a separate OB-GYN residency. Since OB-GYN residency programs are four years in length, this meant that senior residents would have to be recruited from existing training programs. What caliber of senior resident would want to leave their established training program to join a brand new residency program for their final year? Since the new state residency would not be familiar with the hospital or its workings, I suggested that we have a least a one-week transition period to benefit patient care. OB-GYN residents from both programs could work together to allow for a smooth passing of the baton. For the first time, I received insight into the intense competition that goes on between medical schools. The administrations of the two medical schools would not consider my recommendation. So, July 1, 1990, arrived. It was a Sunday, but Labor and Delivery was quite busy. I made rounds with the both teams of residents. Beads of sweat began to appear on the brow of the new state chief OB-GYN resident as the patient presentations continue to increase in number. He furiously scribbled notes on a small paper pad regarding each patient's history.

"Sorry," I said. "This is not how I would have done it. Please take care of our patients."

We transported only one patient to the new southern city hospital that day. She had sickle cell anemia; there was no readily available blood for transfusion and she was *septic* (infection in her bloodstream). I thought it was the least I could do for the new resident team. Just before we left the hospital for the last time, I asked the hospital operator to patch me through to the entire hospital PA system.

"Elvis is leaving the building," I announced.

13

Obstetrics Comes Home

Perhaps the most difficult thing to handle in medicine involves situations when one of your own family needs healthcare. This is even more challenging when it is in the field where you work every day.

Karen and I married in the late spring of my final year of OB-GYN residency. She conceived soon after I graduated from residency. Just before we moved, Karen developed a sore throat with strep. She was fairly miserable.

"One shot of penicillin is all you need," I advised her.

"You must be kidding. You know how much I am scared of needles," she replied.

I managed to get her some samples of an oral antibiotic and her symptoms resolved over the next few days. In those days, low-dose birth control pills were just coming on the market. Rumor had it that taking oral antibiotics could interfere with their protective effect but as residents we thought this was only theoretical. Little did I know! We had planned to wait a few years to start a family. Karen had wanted to apply to midwifery school and I would be a fellow in training with a limited salary. Things have a funny way of working themselves out despite the best of plans.

I was out of town at a research meeting in late July when Karen called. "Guess what, I'm pregnant," she said on the phone.

"Well, that's great," I responded with limited enthusiasm. After all we had planned on starting a family a little later in our marriage. Karen had actually been accepted to midwifery school at the medical school.

We became the talk of the town back at my OB-GYN residency program. When the pharmaceutical rep talked with my former junior residents they would say, "Yeh, that's a great pill you have. Our last chief resident's wife conceived on it," they pointed out.

After hearing this multiple times, the rep finally contacted me to verify that Karen was indeed pregnant. She asked me to file an *adverse reaction* report with the FDA.

I asked Bill, my partner, to care for Karen during the pregnancy. After all, he was the best clinician I knew. Bill was not as touchy, feely as Karen would have liked.

At about four months into the pregnancy, Karen had a routine blood test drawn called *alpha-fetoprotein*. Originally the test was designed to detect fetuses with spina bifida. A high level meant that the fetus might have this condition. A study published that same year suggested that a low level was associated with a fetus with *Down syndrome (trisomy 21)*[43]. Dr. Wood offered us an amniocentesis to check our unborn daughter's chromosomes (*the twenty-three pairs of DNA that provide our inheritance*). He performed the procedure with ease, although Karen later told me he missed the spot where he had injected the numbing medicine into her skin when he placed the larger needle to remove a sample of fluid from around the fetus.

An anxious week passed, then I called the cytogenetics lab. "We won't have a final result until another week," they told me.

"I just need to know that there are only two not three chromosome number 21s," I replied.

"There are two," said the lab tech. This meant that the result was normal. We breathed a sigh of relief. The rest of the pregnancy passed uneventfully.

Karen was working in the Labor and Delivery unit at the private hospital as an OB nurse until the night before she went into labor. The shared coffee pot for the unit was located in the nurses' lounge. The rule was when the door to the lounge was closed, the nurses were changing into scrubs.

One day, Dr .Wood, now Karen's obstetrician, barged through the closed door of the nurses' lounge while Karen was changing clothes. He went straight to the coffee pot and poured himself a steaming Styrofoam cup of black coffee. Without a word, he turned and exited the room.

A few seconds later, he returned to face Karen. "My wife wears those same kind of panties," he declared. That was Bill, always a man of few words!

A few weeks later, at around 6 a.m., Karen shook me awake.

"I think I am in labor," she said. "I've been contracting since three this morning. We headed off to the same hospital where we both worked.

Karen had handpicked her OB nurse to care for her in labor. Soon after she arrived to Labor and Delivery, the nurse put her on the fetal monitor but she was having problems getting a good recording. She tried to place a *scalp electrode* (a little spiral wire that goes just under the skin of the scalp on the top of the baby's head to record the heartbeat) but struggled with it for a while. She was nervous – here was one of her fellow nurses in labor and her husband was a MFM fellow to boot.

Karen looked at me, "Can you just put it on for me?" she asked.

I placed the electrode.

Karen had enlisted a physician to be her *Doula*. The definition of a *Doula* is a person, usually a woman, who is not medically trained but who gives help and support to a woman during the birth of her baby[44]. Its literal translation is "one who mothers the mother." Clearly, Karen's Doula was a step above—Dr. Haynes was a board-certified MFM specialist. Karen had cared for many of this physician's patients in labor and she liked the way she coached them. Karen really wanted to try natural childbirth. With each contraction, she would start moaning with discomfort. It was a hard thing for me to sit by and watch while doing nothing. A moistened wash towel to the forehead was not much help.

Finally at five centimeters of dilation, she acquiesced and agreed it was time for an epidural. The anesthesiologist arrived to our labor room and started asking the usual questions—allergies, medical problems, etc. At that point, Karen had removed her hospital gown and was sitting nude on the labor bed ready for the epidural to be placed.

"I have no medical problems and no allergies. Let's just get this done," she told the anesthesiologist.

He did not realize that he knew Karen as one of the Labor and Delivery nurses who had worked on the very same OB unit. He walked around the bed to see who he was addressing and became embarrassed when he realized who this nude woman was. The epidural took the edge off even though it seemed to work well on only one side of her body.

It finally came time for the delivery. Much to Dr. Wood's chagrin, Dr. Haynes decided to assist him with the delivery. Rachael was born into this world with the guidance of four hands from two MFM specialists guiding her head.

As one of the many gifts we received at our wedding, one of my dad's business partners had sent us a case of Dom Perignon champagne. After the ceremony, the wedding party managed to partake of nine of the bottles but we decided to save three for special events later in our life. Clearly a first birth qualified as such an event, so we uncorked a bottle with our supper later that evening.

Our second child, Kaitlyn, was more of a planned event. Karen had decided not to come back to work as a Labor and Delivery nurse and instead to stay home to be a mom to Rachael. On Fridays, Karen would come into my office to help with ultrasounds and procedures on private patients.

On one particular Friday when she was pregnant with Kaitlyn, we had a patient cancellation. When I turned around, Karen was lying on the examination table.

"Let's just go ahead and do an amnio to check the chromosomes. I want you to do it. I have seen how well you do this," she told me.

As a general rule, the medical profession frowns upon a physician caring for his own family members. This is an unwritten code that most of us follow. Occasionally we will call in a prescription for an antibiotic but performing a procedure on a family member is pretty much taboo.

An *amniocentesis* is an outpatient procedure usually done in an office setting. A needle is used to take a sample of amniotic fluid from around the fetus. Ultrasound is used throughout the procedure to make sure the needle does not injure the fetus on first entry. The risk for loss of the pregnancy is often quoted as one in 200 cases. In truth in experienced hands, the risk pf pregnancy loss may be closer to one in 1000 cases[45]. In the past, amniocentesis was offered to every woman over age thirty-five since they were considered *advanced maternal age* and were at higher risk for *Down syndrome*. At the time of their birth, female infants are born with her entire complement of all the eggs in their ovaries they will ever produce in their lifetime. Some of the eggs are depleted through monthly ovulation and some regress spontaneously. When the ovaries run out of eggs, menopause begins. The older the eggs get in the ovaries, the higher the chance that the chromosomes will not divide correctly once the egg is fertilized by a sperm. This process is called *non-disjunction* and leads to *trisomy 21* or *Down syndrome*. However, since younger women make up more of the pregnant population at any one time, there are actually more children born to women under the age of thirty-five than to those born to women who are greater than thirty-five years of age. For a time, all pregnant women were screened for *Down syndrome* in the second trimester looking for subtle ultrasound findings such as how thick the fetal tissue was behind the neck[46]. In addition, several other blood tests were added to the original alpha-fetoprotein blood test to create a *triple or quad screen* to detect *Down syndrome*[47]. Then British investigators determined that if a first trimester fetus was seen on ultrasound to have an enlarged clear space behind its neck (*nuchal translucency*), there was a significant risk for *Down syndrome*[48]. Finally, today, the field of prenatal genetic screening has advanced to the point that DNA from the placenta can be found in a blood sample from the pregnant patient[49]. This can then be analyzed to detect several different fetal chromosomal abnormalities. Non-invasive prenatal testing (*NIPT*) is now offered to almost all pregnant patients in most developed countries to check for *Down syndrome*. The very name of the test (probably conceived by smart marketing folks) implies that amniocentesis is invasive and therefore dangerous to the fetus. As a result, pregnant women now shy away from amniocentesis and decide that *NIPT* is accurate enough to check for *Down syndrome*. Clearly this is not the case since an *NIPT* test in a younger patient has a higher rate of being a false positive result. In all positive *NIPT* cases, an amniocentesis or chorion villus biopsy is indicated to check the actual fetal chromosomes.

NIPT testing was not available when Karen was pregnant. I took a deep breath and easily guided the needle into the fluid-filled space that surrounded our unborn Kaitlyn. Her chromosome results later came back normal.

This time things were a little more calm around our second delivery. This time Karen's waters broke while she was at home.

We were having the living room at our house painted at the time. Michael was a good painter but he was slow to complete the job.

Karen emerged from the bathroom. "Michael, I'm going to have a baby today," she said. "You'd better have this painting done by the time I get home with this new baby." He looked at her in disbelief!

As fortune would have it, I was at the hospital with one of my own patients that was in labor. A colleague's former co-fellow's wife, Peggy, brought Karen to the hospital and kept Racheal for us. This would be the first time Rachael would be separated from her mother since her birth two years earlier.

After arriving to Labor and Delivery, the belts of the fetal monitors were attached. The baby looked good and there were no contractions. Usually in these situations, the OB has two options - have the patient walk around a bit to see if labor will start on its own or go ahead and induce labor with oxytocin We chose the more conservative route. I had yet to make my evening rounds on my patients in the hospital so Karen and I decided to do them together. As I entered each of my patients' rooms, I would introduce Karen.

"This is my wife. She's helping me out on rounds today. We're trying to see if we can get her to go into labor," I declared much to their amazement.

Labor contractions finally started a few hours later. Karen had picked Dr. Haynes, her previous Doula, to be her obstetrician for this delivery. No epidural was needed this time as labor was much shorter. Karen pushed three times and Kaitlyn was born into this world.

Most OB patients only stay in the hospital for one to two days after a vaginal delivery. I decided to have Karen stay on the sixth floor postoperative unit at the hospital instead of the usual postpartum floor. The unit was set aside for the VIP patients. It was going to cost me a few extra dollars for the difference in the room rate but I thought she deserved it. After all, I was an attending physician now, so my salary was a bit better than when I was a fellow. The rooms were twice as large as the usual postpartum room and a newspaper of your choice was delivered each morning. Extra special was the little lady with a lace apron who came by mid-morning and mid-afternoon with a cart of crackers and a selection of cheeses! Karen's delivery did not occur until around 3 a.m. so we were both exhausted when we finally arrived in the room.

Then there was a knock on the door at around 5 a.m. It was the charge nurse for the floor.

"I really hate to disturb you, but the nurses on Labor and Delivery called wondering if you would mind coming down," she said. "They have some sort of emergency and there are no other OB doctors in the hospital."

I was sleeping in scrubs so I did not have to change. Adrenaline was coursing through my veins as I jumped up and ran down the three flights of stairs to the Labor and Delivery Unit.

"They need you in room six," the clerk informed me as I ran to the nursing station.

I entered the room to find three nurses frantically trying to calm a pregnant patient.

"She's 28 weeks pregnant and completely dilated," the head nurse informed me. "There are two feet coming out of the vagina."

I quickly donned a pair of gloves and examined the patient. She was right, the fetus was a *double footling* breech with its buttocks descended to her mother's vaginal opening. She was right, the fetus was a double footling breech with its buttocks descended to her mother's vaginal opening.

"PUSH," I instructed.

Out popped this little body and then the head. The neonatologist whisked the baby away to the warmer for some oxygen. A few minutes later the little girl was headed to the NICU. Her mom looked at me with tears in her eyes.

"Thank you for being here for us," she said.

After a few hours of much needed sleep, I wrapped up Kaitlyn and carried her over to my office. After all it was on the same floor of the hospital, so who would miss her. Our secretaries were delighted to meet her. Later that night, Karen and I opened our second bottle of Dom Perignon to celebrate. We went home the next day.

When we conceived our third child, Karen let me pick the name after the ultrasound showed it was a girl. I chose Erin, the namesake of a recent medical student that had been an amazing attribute to our

OB service during her elective rotation. The pregnancy was uneventful until it was time for delivery.

Contractions started on Christmas Eve. Karen had no intention in delivering a baby on Christmas day. In years past, intravenous alcohol was used to treat premature uterine contractions some years earlier. Patients were later given an oral shot of vodka every six hours once they were transferred to the floor. Today we use other medications to stop premature contractions like *terbutaline, indomethacin,* or intravenous *magnesium sulfate.* Having worked in a hospital that used alcohol to stop contractions, Karen thought it was worth a try. Half a bottle of wine later, her contractions had subsided.

It was now the day before New Year's Eve. Labor contractions had begun in earnest. Dr. Haynes' midwife came to the house to check on Karen and she was eight centimeters dilated. I again had to arrange coverage, since I was at the hospital with one of my own private patients who was in labor.

"I think I am going to stay home and deliver in the bathtub," Karen informed the midwife.

"Your husband will never forgive me," she replied. A few minutes later they headed into the hospital.

In fact, more recent data has raised concern regarding the safety of home deliveries[50]. Newborn babies are twice as likely to have seizures if they are born at home as compared to a hospital.

Dr. Haynes was out of town, so her partner, Dr. Liz Snipe, would have to deliver Karen. I liked Liz. She was a self-made woman. Earlier in life she had been a long-distance truck driver and then had decided to go to medical school. She was older and more mature than most of the other private OB attendings. The only problem was that she lived almost sixty miles away and this was our third baby. As a general rule, labor gets shorter with each successive pregnancy.

"I'll get someone to stand by for you if you can't get here on time," I told her.

"No problem. I'll be there in about an hour," she responded.

Karen was completely dilated when Liz arrived.

Liz looked up at me, "Do you want to deliver this one since it is going to be your last?"

I pondered the proposal for a moment and then thought, what the heck this would be special. As Karen began to push, Liz began to instruct me on the proper technique for performing a vaginal delivery.

"I think I have this," I responded. "I have a vested interest here as this is my wife and my daughter."

Karen reared up on her elbows in the labor bed between contractions, "Will you two stop arguing and get this baby out of me!"

I delivered Erin easily. This gorgeous little girl looked up at me through blue eyes. We had a special bond.

At many subsequent holiday dinners, Erin would brag to her two older sisters on several occasions, "Daddy delivered me, but not either one of you." Erin would go on to be the only one of my three daughters to enter medicine. After graduation from Physician Associate school in the midst of the COVID pandemic, she would have great difficulty in finding a job. After volunteering in my office for a period of time, we would come to hire her to work by my side each day.

We only had three bottles of Dom Perignon saved from our wedding so we decided that Erin would be the last addition to our growing family. My wife and I had envisioned a family of four children. I decided if the next pregnancy resulted in a girl, it would be time to stop. After all there would be expenses like proms, college, and weddings. As the oldest of five boys in my family, I worked summers as a carpenter and an offshore oil company's cook's helper to pay for my own car insurance and half of my college and medical school tuition and living expenses. I would not have the same expectation for our daughters.

Karen underwent a tubal ligation the next day. That night I picked up a steak dinner and we celebrated with the last bottle of champagne. It was New Year's Eve and Karen was fast asleep. One of my former OB-GYN residents who was now a new attending, came by to say hello.

"Say, if you have a moment, can I ask you to look at a patient with me?", she asked.

"Sure," I responded. "Karen is asleep."

We went to a postpartum room to examine her patient. Her vaginal delivery had been eventful, but the nurses had called to say the patient was experiencing a new onset of pain in her vagina.

"I found a small hematoma when I examined her earlier," my colleague said.

"Well let's have a peek," I responded. With the help of a penlight I was able to see that the hematoma was now about the size of a grapefruit.

"We need to take her to surgery," I recommended.

"Can you assist?' came the reply. "I've not done one of these this big before."

An hour later, the patient was asleep in surgery. We opened up the inside wall of the vagina and evacuated the clots. We sutured the bleeders and placed a pack.

The New Year arrived a few minutes later.

14

New Digs

Our new hospital was never short of challenging cases. We had only been there one week when our OB service was called urgently to the *surgical intensive care unit (SICU)*. A young woman who appeared to be around twenty years of age had been admitted to the emergency room with a gunshot wound to her head. Her admitting laboratory tests had just returned with a positive pregnancy test. Upon the OB team's arrival, it was clear that the patient was visibly pregnant as evidenced by the protuberance in her abdomen. We of course had no way of knowing exactly how far along the patient was in her pregnancy.

Without immediate access to an ultrasound in the ICU, we measured our patient's fundal height to be twenty-four centimers. We assumed that the patient was therefore 24 weeks into the pregnancy. Even today with all the modern technical advances in neonatal intensive care, 24 weeks gestation is considered the threshold when a fetus can survive outside of the womb. About 50% of babies at this gestation will survive; 30% or more will have long-term developmental problems like blindness or seizures. Faced with a decision where the fetus might be viable, we elected to proceed with an emergency C-section.

As were discussing plans for moving the patient to the new Labor and Delivery operating rooms, the nurse interrupted, "Her blood pressure is falling. It's now 60 over 40. And falling."

"No time to move her," I said. "Can someone get me a scalpel?"

"You can't do this in the ICU!" her nurse told me.

"That's the only way we are going to get a baby from this dying women," I replied.

Someone handed me a number ten blade scalpel and I proceed with a *perimortem C-section* in the ICU bed. The baby was delivered thirty seconds later. The neonatal team had been called so they were standing nearby to take the baby. As I delivered this little girl, I could see that her eyelids were still fused shut. Like newborn puppies, the eyelids of the human fetus remained fused until about 25½ weeks of gestation. The neonatologist put a breathing tube down the baby's throat and whisked it off to the nursery. Unfortunately, she died three days later. After the delivery, the patient's blood pressure recovered to a normal level. This was not surprising since the blood that remains in the uterus after the baby is born gets infused into the patient's bloodstream when the womb contracts down. We sutured the patient's womb and skin together at the bedside. She died from her head injury two hours later.

Most women believe that pregnancy lasts nine months. In truth, a patient's normal due date is 40 weeks after the first day of patient's last menstrual period. This date was once called the *estimated date of confinement (EDC)*. When most obstetrical deliveries occurred in the home, women were confined to bedrest at their home by this date. Today the term *EDC* has been replaced with *EDD, the estimated date of delivery.* This is probably a kinder, gentler term since we no longer confine women to bed at the end of their pregnancy. In truth only 4% of women deliver on this projected date; 70% deliver in a window of ten days earlier or later than when they are "due." Deliveries that occur prior to 37 weeks gestation are called *premature* and those that occur after 41 weeks are called *post-dates.*

The average woman ovulates two weeks before the onset of pregnancy; fertilization occurs in the far end of the fallopian tube soon thereafter. So, pregnancy is actually 38 weeks in length. Even more confusing is the breakdown of *trimesters* (derived from Latin for three months) of pregnancy. The first *trimester* is twelve weeks long and the third *trimester* begins at 28 weeks. This makes the second *trimester* sixteen weeks in length—confusing to all. Ultrasound has become the main method of dating pregnancies today. Prior to the widespread use of ultrasound, clinical examination was the main way that an OB-GYN confirmed the length of a gestation. When a pregnancy reaches the fifth month (twenty weeks out of the total of forty weeks), the top of the uterus can be felt at about the level of a woman's navel. After that, one can measure the *fundal height* (the distance in centimeters from the pubic bone to the top of the uterus), and in most cases, the number of centimeters equals the number of weeks of gestation. Despite the almost universal use of ultrasound to date pregnancies and watch for fetal growth problems, OB-GYN's still measure the fundal height at each prenatal visit. Perhaps it is our compulsiveness as physicians that forces us to fill in this blank in the *electronic medical record (EMR).*

One of the most difficult situations that an OB-GYN will face is dealing with a patient that is of the Jehovah Witness faith. These individuals refuse blood and its components even if it means their death. This practice is based on a passage from the Old Testament of the Bible. Genesis 9:4 states: "God allowed Noah and his family to add animal flesh to their diet after the flood but commanded them not to eat the blood. God told Noah; "Only flesh with its soul—its blood you must not eat." Jehovah Witnesses feel that since all mankind are descendants of Noah, the rule applies to all. Administering blood to a Jehovah Witness patient can result in their damnation to hell after their death.

This poses significant ethical issues for the physician who is sworn to save patients. Some will honor the patient's wishes and allow them to die. Others (including myself) will not. Even more challenging is a situation where the patient is still pregnant and a blood transfusion may save her life and the life of her unborn child. In these cases, judges have ordered the patient to receive the transfusion until she has delivered since the fetus has not had the opportunity to decide if he/she believes in the same religious principles as its mother. Other legal guidance on the issue is confusing. Administration of blood can result in assault and battery charges being filed against the physician—a misdemeanor crime. A decision not to give blood and to allow the patient to die has resulted in malpractice litigation cases brought by surviving family members. Jury awards in these cases were based on the family's claim that they would have allowed the transfusion if the physician had properly explained the serious nature of the situation.

My mentor, Dr. Bogs, was often heard to say, "Transfuse the patient and put my name on the chart as the attending. I want to be on the front page of the city newspaper as saving the patient's life."

When I was seeing private OB patients in my earlier years as an attending, I was sure to ask them at the very first prenatal visit if they would accept blood if this was needed in their pregnancy. On one occasion, a patient informed me she was a Jehovah Witness and would not.

"Then I must tell you that I will transfuse you if I believe it will prevent you from dying."

She told me she could not accept this. We both decided it would be better for her to seek care from another OB.

Of course, when I was the attending at the inner-city hospital, I had to supervise the care of whatever patient was admitted. On one occasion, the patient was only 12 weeks pregnant. She had seen a midwife in her prenatal clinic. The midwife used a new device called a *Cytobrush* to perform a pap smear. Historically, the pap smear was usually undertaken with a wooden spatula to scrape cells from the outside of the cervix to look for early cancer cells. A moistened Q tip was then gently placed in the cervical canal leading to the uterus to obtain *endocervical cells* to be sure there is no cancerous lesion located higher up. The *Cytobrush* had been recently introduced as a better way to obtain an adequate sample of *endocervical cells*. In this case however, the midwife, new to the use of the *Cytobrush*, had advanced it too far into the cervical canal, causing the patient to begin bleeding from her placenta which, in this case, was located in the lower portion of the patient's womb.

I was called to the operating room after the patient had been transferred from the clinic with profuse vaginal bleeding. When I arrived, the patient was asleep with general anesthesia with a breathing tube in place. The chief resident had decided that the only way to stop the bleeding was to undertake a *dilation and curettage (D&C)* to end the pregnancy.

"Oh, by the way," she informed me. "She is a Jehovah Witness."

Even though there was evidence of a fetal heart beat on ultrasound, I agreed that the only way to stop the bleeding was to remove the fetus and the placenta. We proceeded with procedure but the bleeding became even heavier. At this point the anesthesiologist looked at me.

"She has lost a lot of blood," she said. "We are beginning to see changes on her EKG tracing. I am worried we may lose her soon."

I took off my gown and gloves and headed to the family waiting rom. There I found the patient's husband with two of the couple's small children.

"Mr. Martinez, we unfortunately had to end your wife's pregnancy to try to stop her bleeding," I informed him. "She continues to bleed despite our best efforts. Normally I would proceed with a hysterectomy but I am concerned that your wife may not survive the surgery. I really need to transfuse her."

"We are Jehovah Witnesses," he said. "We are not allowed to accept blood."

"I know that, but without blood, your wife will die and you will be raising these two children," I replied.

"Go ahead and give her blood doc if you think you can save her life. But don't tell her that I told you to do that."

A few minutes later, we transfused the patient with red blood cells while we packed her uterus with gauze. Several units of blood and plasma later, the bleeding stopped. The next day, I called my risk management office at the medical school to ask for advice.

"The patient's husband does not want me to tell his wife that we gave her blood," I said.

"You have to inform her of your decision. It is her right," was the response.

I knew in my heart that was the best course. Several days later, I called for a family meeting. The patient, her husband, and a Jehovah Witness elder attended.

"You were asleep," I told the patient. "I had to talk to your husband to help make a decision on giving you blood. He made a difficult decision to allow you to survive to care for your two children."

"He should not have let you to do that," she responded glaring at her husband.

The elder interjected, "Because you were asleep and did not consciously make a decision to accept blood, you will remain a member of the faith."

Medicine is a complex specialty. Many times there are several options to treat a particular clinical situation. A breast cancer might be treated by a *mastectomy* (removal of the entire breast) or a more conservative approach can be taken with a localized *wedge resection* of the tumor followed by radiation. Who decides—the patient or her physician? In the past, it was always the physician. After all, he/she has the most experience with the disease. When one has squeaky brakes on a car, do we go to the mechanic's shop and start asking for all the options of what can be done? Or do we leave the car and trust the mechanic to solve the problem? But in the last decade, there has been a paradigm shift in medicine. Now instead of making the best decision for the patient, the physician is relegated to presenting all the options with their associated risks and benefits. Many of my cases involve the difficult decision as to whether to continue a pregnancy that is complicated by a severe birth defect in the fetus.

Often, I am asked, "If it was your wife what would you do?"

I find myself saying, "It's really not fair to you to tell you what I might recommend for my family. You and your wife need to weigh the various options and decide for yourself whether this fits with your religious and moral beliefs."

Sometimes I think the patient really wants us to make the decision. After all, the statistics can be confusing to even the most learned of individuals. In times of emergencies, however, this new paradigm of shared decision-making reverts to that of previous days. Take the case of a patient in labor who begins to experience fetal distress. The fetal monitor attached to the patient's abdomen may be showing a very slow heart rate. Without prompt delivery, the placenta will deliver insufficient oxygen to the fetus, causing death or severe disability. The patient may be advanced enough in labor that a forceps delivery would be possible. In other situations, the younger physician may not feel comfortable attempting forceps and will want to proceed with an emergency C-section.

And so the scene normally plays out with the physician informing the patient, "Ms. X, your baby is showing signs of severe fetal distress. We need to move quickly and perform an emergency C-section."

"Whatever you think best," is the typical response.

Obviously in an emergency situation, there is no time for discussing many options. The patient trusts the physician to make the best decision. In the case of non-emergent situations, I still believe there can be times when the physician can express his/her opinion as to the best course of action.

Physicians learn from their mistakes. Today we call these *near misses*—a kinder, gentler term used these days. There are two major processes for evaluating these errors. The time-honored approach is the *morbidity and mortality (M&M)* conference. In this scenario, residents in training are asked to present cases that resulted in unanticipated medical complications in patient care. In the worse-case scenario, this may have led to the patient's (or her baby's) untimely death. Cases at our institution were picked by the chief OB resident and the most senior resident on the team that cared for the patient presented the specifics of the case. M&M was held weekly and most of the full-time faculty attended. It was held in a large auditorium, with the resident presenting from a lonely podium in the front. For the residents, it was probably the most intimidating experience of their training. Not that it had to be, but several of our faculty were known for their brash mannerisms of calling residents out on their judgements that had not gone well. A favorite ploy of the more prepared resident was to get the faculty arguing with one another on a particular point. In the later years of M&M, we decided to assign a specific faculty member to proctor the meeting in an effort to keep order. This proved to be only partially successful.

The second process for review was called the *Quality Assurance (QA) committee*. In its original format, the OB-GYN department would develop a list of quality indicators, some of which were proposed by national organizations. Individual patient cases would be brought to the committee's attention for *peer-review* (a review by physicians of the same specialty). If there was felt to be a deviation from the *standard of care*, the committee chair would send a letter to the individual private physician (or supervising faculty member in the case of a resident case) and ask for a response. The response letter was then reviewed by the committee to see if any further corrective action was needed.

Hopefully, a review process like this could prevent the recent case of "Dr. Death"—a neurosurgeon named Christopher Duntsch who was sentenced to life in prison for causing major injury to multiple patients and the death of two patients[51]. This physician completed an MD, PhD program at the University of Tennessee at Memphis medical school. Residency training in neurosurgery at the same institution was followed by a prestigious one-year fellowship in minimal invasive neurosurgery. During his residency, there were documented issues with his cocaine abuse. Dr. Duntsch used his PhD training to create several start-up biotech companies, but when funding for these dried up, he returned to clinical care. He moved to Texas in 2011 and joined a neurosurgical practice in the Plano area. Calls to his training programs verified his credentials and lack of behavioral problems. Then he began to have devastating surgical outcomes including several patient deaths. A later investigation revealed that the hospital had decided that his surgeries should be proctored by another surgeon; however, this was not undertaken. After losing clinical privileges at the first hospital, he was credentialed at a second institution in Dallas. A letter from the administrator at the original hospital stated that he had left in good standing. Due to continued poor outcomes, his medical license was finally revoked by the Texas Medical Board in 2013. Criminal charges were brought against him for aggravated assault, and after a jury trial, he was convicted and sentenced to life in prison.

Although there is obviously still a place for the review of individual physician outcomes, today's quality assurance programs concentrate on systematic issues. Organizations like *The Leapfrog Group* or *The Joint Commission* provide core or quality indicators for a particular specialty to track. A hospital's statistics are then judged against those of similar hospitals. In obstetrics, today's typical indicators include items like how many patients in premature labor get steroids to help accelerate their premature baby's lung function and the number of patients that have their labor induced prior to 37 weeks gestation (considered as the time when the baby's lungs are mature) without a clear medical indication.

These processes are important for improving the quality of our health care. A 2000 study conducted by the Institute of Medicine entitled *To Err is Human* concluded that death from medical errors is the third leading cause of death in the United States[52]. It's estimated that 98,000 lives are lost each year—the equivalent to a Boeing 747 jet crashing with no survivors every two and a half days. During recent times, two newly designed Boeing 737 Max 8 jet aircrafts crashed in less than six months, killing 157 and 189 individuals. After the second crash, nations around the world grounded all of these 737's until investigators could decide if there was a design flaw[53]. So why has there not been more of a public outcry regarding preventable deaths due to medical mistakes? One can only suppose that since the problem occurs slowly and is poorly covered by the news media that it does not draw much attention.

Obstetrical admissions are no less immune to issues with patient safety—in this case two individuals are affected, the mother and her baby. Complications during delivery such as birth trauma are 6% higher on weekends when staffing is decreased[54].

After we moved to our new obstetrical hospital, another attending, Dr. Hankins, and I decided to form a quality assurance (QA) committee for peer review of obstetrical outcomes. At our request, we were formally appointed as co-chairs of the committee by the Chairman of the OB-GYN department. Quality indicators for patient care were chosen based on recommendations from our national college— *The American College of Obstetricians and Gynecologists*. One particular physician came under our intense scrutiny by our newly formed committee. Dr. Wienman was a MD, PhD. I have a theory about these physicians based on my experiences with at least a dozen of these individuals throughout my career. As a general rule, they turn out to be poor clinicians. What is interesting is that these very intelligent individuals normally achieve their PhD degree first, followed by their MD degree. Yet they reverse the order of their degrees at the end of their name. Perhaps they believe that the MD title is more prestigious. The mind of the PhD is wired differently—it is driven by data and research outcomes. I hypothesize that once these individuals complete their PhD training they soon realize the financial ceiling of their career path (a PhD makes approximately one-third

the annual salary of an MD). Often exposed to the medical community, they realize that they are smart enough to survive the rigors of
medical school with the possibility of enhanced future income. And
yet their brains are not wired for clinical problem solving or manual
dexterity as a surgeon.

Dr. Wienman was obviously a very bright individual. His PhD
was in physiology (the study of how living organisms work). He had
then gone on to medical school followed by residencies in internal
medicine and OB-GYN, then fellowship training in MFM at prestigious West Coast schools. His recruitment involved start-up funding
to develop a sheep lab for research in pregnancy. Soon after Dr. Wienman's arrival, it became apparent that he was not comfortable in the
intense clinical setting of our inner-city hospital. Several cases began
to come under review where the quality of the patient's care was
questionable when he served as the attending faculty for supervision
on the resident teaching service. Letters of inquiry were generated
from the committee with copies to the Chairman of the department.
At some point, Dr. Wienman elected to leave the institution and seek
employment at another medical school. He received an initial job
offer that was retracted once the institution did its due diligence and
made phone inquiries. To this day, I am not sure who answered these
inquiries; my opinion was never requested.

Dr. Wienman filed a slander lawsuit against the medical school
naming both myself and my co-chair of the QA committee as the
likely culprits of his poor references. The school decided that they
would provide our legal counsel; however, we would have to release
the proceedings of the QA committee. In our state, these are considered protected, so that physicians can feel free to discuss these cases
without fear of reprisal. My co-chair, Dr. Hankins, and I decided we
would not release our files. If we were required to do so, we threatened to be hostile witnesses for our own medical school. In the end

the attorneys had their way since they decided the co-chairs did not own the minutes of the QA meetings—they were ruled the property of the medical school. The specific letters to Dr. Wienman were obtained and actually send out for external review "to be sure we were doing things right." Depositions followed. Mine lasted three straight days, eight hours each day. Dr. Wienman sat on the plaintiff's side of the table glaring at me the entire time.

All aspects of the department were fair game. At one point, Dr. Wienman's attorney inquired as to whether Dr. Winkle (the Director of the MFM Division) was an alcoholic. This upset me tremendously as I felt it had no bearing on the case.

"Can I ask for a break?" I asked. A few minutes later I was in the bathroom conferring with my attorney.

"What does this have to do with this case?" I asked. "I don't want this in the public record."

"You will have to answer," he instructed me. "Or he can take you in front of the judge to get an answer," he responded.

Not what I wanted to hear. We were back on the record at the deposition.

"Dr. when we left for the break, I was asking you if Dr. Winkle was an alcoholic."

"Yes, I remember," I responded planning my strategy. "Counselor, I am a board-certified Maternal-Fetal Medicine specialist," I said. "Substance abuse with alcohol is a *DSMIII* diagnosis (this is the list of categories of psychiatric diseases that psychiatrists use to classify their patients).

"Answer my question. Is Dr. Winkle an alcoholic?" he repeated.

"I've already given you an answer," I responded.

"Answer my question or I will take you in front of the judge," he threatened.

"Take me to the pope and I will give him the same answer," I responded.

The deposition ended shortly thereafter. I understand that the deposition of my co-chair was equally dramatic, although our attorneys told us we were not allowed to discuss the specific details with one another. Our school attorneys were faced with a dilemma—either the QA committee and it chairs were correct and Dr. Wienman should have been removed from clinical service by the Chairman of the department OR the Chairman of the department should have directed the misguided attempts of the QA committee to cease and desist. When all the dust settled, the lawyers got together and settled the case for an undisclosed amount of money. I am told that the funds were sufficient enough that Dr. Wienman retired never to see patients again. I guess this was a small consolation for the efforts the QA committee had put forth. Interestingly, I recently noted on the state website that he stills maintains his medical license. Soon after the incident, Dr. Hankins and I decided to disband the QA committee. We did not want to see the careers of its other members placed in jeopardy. Our experience was traumatic enough!

Dr. Winkle had taken over the MFM fellowship Directorship with the departure of Dr. Bale. Since I was involved with teaching the current MFM fellows almost on a daily basis, he thought it appropriate to name me the fellowship Director. The only obstacle was my age. Seems at thirty-five years of age, I was eligible to run for the Presidency of the United States, but in the eyes of the *ABOG*, the certifying body for the fellowships, I did not have the five years of experience needed to qualify as the fellowship Director. In any event, I was named the assistant Director and one year later was promoted to the Director. Foreign medical graduates who come to the U.S. for training are motivated individuals. Many have completed residency training in their native countries but the U.S. requires them to repeat clinical training here in order to eventually be recognized as board certified in their specialty. In these years, our fellowship program was lucky enough to recruit individuals from South Africa, Lebanon, and Belgium. The South African fellow presented a dilemma. He had been promised a combined OB-GYN residency / MFM fellowship position on an abbreviated schedule by Dr. Bale prior to his departure from our department. The second wrinkle was that Dr. Fugue was from a country actively involved in apartheid. Our residency Director was African-American. Dr. Point would not make it easy for the transition. Dr. Fugue arrived to our program in August with his wife and a newborn baby in tow. He was informed that he would need to complete both the third and fourth years of the OB-GYN residency "like everyone else." This also meant that he would have to take every other night of in-house call in August to make up for the missed call nights in July. Dr. Fugue's career and my career would come to cross again later in our lives.

ABOG states that one of the primary roles for the fellowship Director is to be sure that the fellow completes a thesis project in the course of their two years of training. This is no easy task, as many fellows arrive with no research experience. I have always questioned the wisdom of this requirement. Some fellows know that they will enter private practice after completing their training. In this scenario, requiring a thesis project seems ludicrous. Perhaps the rationale is that this teaches the individual an appreciation for medical research. Most MFM fellowships are sponsored by medical schools. In my opinion, the more likely reason for the *ABOG* research requirement is to enable continued research productivity from a department of OB-GYN. In any event, ABOG placed a significant emphasis on the

Director's role in assuring the fellow accomplished this research. I would usually meet with the new fellows at the start of the academic year and suggest a few possibilities for research endeavors. Many times the fellow would develop their own interest and come to me with an innovative idea. These were always the best projects. Often, they led to enhanced knowledge for me as well as the fellow.

One particular project stands out as such an example. Dr. Sherm was a German physician who had immigrated to the U.S. and completed an OB-GYN residency here. He came to my office one day with an idea.

"I want to study the effects of airline travel on pregnancy," he said.

"Interesting," I replied. "Have you done a literature search to see what has been published?" I asked.

"Not really much out there. Just some studies in sheep taken up to the top of a mountain in a van," he answered.

"Have at it. Let me know what you come up with for a research design."

Dr. Sherm first approached a local commercial airline based out of our city. He suggested that they allow him to put a patient in the back on a short flight and he would bring in an ultrasound machine to study the fetus during the flight. The airline of course thought he was joking.

"Not going to happen," they responded.

Then he found a hyperbaric oxygen chamber at a local medical school that had been outfitted by *NASA* to study the effects of altitude. He proposed a study of pregnant rabbits to see the effects of a simulated trans-Atlantic airline flight on their fetuses. This sounded like a feasible project. The chamber was about eight feet round and twenty feet long. An air lock at one end allowed one to go in an out even when the chamber was at "high altitude." The study required us to unbolt the large door off the end of the chamber to wheel in the ultrasound machine and the conditions would be a bit crowded with rabbit cages and three or four folks to help with the blood collections. I found the funds we needed to pay the pump tech to run the chamber for the experiment. The most interesting part of the whole endeavor was that we were actually part of the experiment since we would be in the chamber with the rabbits.

There were only two glitches. We had to be out of the chamber by 7 a.m. The same facility housed a second *hyperbaric oxygen chamber* that was used by patients for special treatments. Seems that patients came from many surrounding states and even other countries to be treated in this chamber. *Hyperbaric oxygen* (think Michael Jackson) is used for the treatment of wounds that are not healing properly. The high levels of the oxygen under pressure are pushed into the patient's tissues to accelerate their natural healing process. The second fly in the ointment came from the research nurses. We would need one of them to help us to manage the blood samples we were obtaining from the rabbit fetuses.

The lead research nurse came to my office. "I have met with all the research nurses and they do not want to help with Dr. Sherm's study," she said.

"What is it? Are you'll concerned about the crammed space," I replied.

"In a sense." She looked at meet sheepishly.

"And?" I asked.

"Well this is awkward, but Dr. Sherm is European you know and well, he doesn't wear deodorant," she said. "We can't see ourselves in that small chamber with him for several hours."

"Got it," I responded. "Let me see what I can do."

I called the fellow to my office. "You've designed a great research project. There is only one small issue that we need to address to move forward," I said. "I am so sorry to have to bring this up. In order for the research nurses to help us, they are requesting a change in your personal hygiene since we will be in close quarters for several hours."

Dr, Sherm turned three shades of red.

"Can we fix this?" I asked.

I needed to say no more. The study would be conducted in four phases. The first would be done at high altitude with the normal decreased amount of oxygen that occurs in a normal airline flight (turns out that the airlines pressurize their cabins to about 8,000 feet and at that altitude one is breathing 16% oxygen instead of the normal 21%.) Then there would be three more phases: at altitude with supplemental oxygen like we breathe every day, at sea level, and finally at sea level with nitrous gas pumped into the chamber to reduce the amount of oxygen the rabbits (and we ourselves) would breathe. Each "trip" would last eight hours to mimic a transatlantic crossing by plane. Rabbits would be placed into the chamber at intervals so they were all exposed to the same length of the flight. At about 3 a.m., I would arrive to assist Dr. Sherm with ultrasound so that we could obtain blood samples from the fetuses to check for the amount of acid in their blood. By 7 a.m., we had to unbolt the door at the end of the chamber, remove the ultrasound machine, mop out the floor, and remove all the rabbits like nothing had ever happened. In total we made about twelve "flights." The one I remember the most was the flight at sea level where nitrous gas was being pumped into the chamber to lower the amount of oxygen we were breathing. I made sure to stop by the all-night doughnut shop on the way in to bring fresh pastries to the chamber pump technician—the guy that kept the oxygen (and nitrous) flowing while we were all locked inside this metal cylinder. The flight took place just before Christmas so we had carols playing on the speakers inside the chamber. The nitrous gas we were using to lower the oxygen for the experiment on that day is the same "laughing gas" the dentist gives you. Needless to say, it was quite a scene—all of us giggling and singing along with the chipmunk carols.

The final analysis of the study would show that both the altitude and the lower oxygen level associated with it can cause acid to build up in the fetuses. This was a unique finding with the possibility of having a major impact on recommendations for prolonged airline travel for pregnant patients. More studies would be need to confirm our findings. Like so many controversial results, Dr. Sherm submitted his thesis to a major OB-GYN journal only to be rejected. The article was eventually accepted and published in an obscure hyperbaric medicine journal.

Most academic institutions have a hierarchy of positions as one advances up the ladder in academic medicine. An entry-level position on joining the medical school faculty is *Assistant Professor*. In some institutions, the entry-level position can be *Clinical Instructor*. After a period of time (usually five years), a Chairman will submit a faculty member to the medical school promotions committee for advancement to the level of *Associate Professor*. A national reputation with letters from peers at other institutions supporting the applicant's promotion is needed. In the past, there were two distinct pathways at this point in one's career. A faculty member who was publishing peer-review papers and obtaining research grants would apply for the *tenure track*. An attending who was mostly doing clinical work for the department would be promoted on the *clinical, non-tenure track*. When promoted, this faculty member would be known as a *Clinical Associate Professor* on the signature line of their letters and on their business cards. Five to ten years would then pass before one could be considered for promotion to *Full Professor, tenure track* or *Clinical Full Professor*. For promotion to *Full Professor, tenure track* one would need letters of support from international peers.

Tenure is an interesting concept in education. In earlier times, university professors were considered employees of their institution and were often terminated by members of the board of trustees without just cause. One such example was that of Edward Ross in 1900[55]. Ross, a professor at Stanford, was outspoken on several issues regarding railroad employment practices. Hearing these controversial ideas, the widow of Leland Stanford, the founder of Stanford University, successfully petitioned the board of directors to have Ross terminated. Later in 1915, two university professors arranged a conference of over 600 of their colleagues to address the issue of tenure. This ultimately resulted in the formation of the American Association of University Professors and the publication of the *Declaration of Principles of Academic Freedom and Tenure*.

The concept of what tenure really means continues to evolve at many medical schools in the U.S. I was once told tenure only means that it will be difficult to fire you but all the Chairman has to pay you is the base salary of an English professor at the main university. Since medical school departments are becoming more dependent on clinical revenues to pay their faculty, even the distinction between *Clinical Associate* and *Associate, tenure track* professors is becoming blurred. In fact, many institutions have dropped the term *Clinical* so there is no clear distinction between the two promotion tracks.

Three years after joining the faculty, I asked our department chair if he would consider supporting my promotion to *Associate Professor* on the *tenure track*. We reviewed by curriculum vitae and I had almost fifty peer-reviewed papers published or "in press." This was no small feat in this short period of time. My days were spent managing a busy clinical service of pregnant women at the inner-city hospital. As a result, I often wrote papers at night once all three of my young daughters and my wife had retired. Many times, I would write until 2 a.m. The promotions committee was willing to consider my application but they wanted to see the acceptance letters from the journal editors for all the articles that were *in press*. After these were provided, they promptly approved my promotion.

Most of the papers I had written involved multiple authors. This is usually the case in academic medicine. The first author usually writes the paper while the last author is considered the *senior author*, the individual providing mentorship for the project. The order of the authors between these two names usually involves a decreasing involvement in a particular project. Through the years I have found that the issue of authorship can become quite contentious. Perhaps this is related to the decreasing commitment of academic faculty to publish peer-reviewed literature and the realization that they will need publications on the curriculum vitae for eventual promotion. In any event, I have found it useful to broach the topic of authorship even at the very start of a research project. In addition, many journals today have set forth specific requirements for authorship confirmed by statements signed by all of the authors when the paper is submitted for review.

On reviewing my CV, I realize that there is only one publication where I am the sole author. During my early years as an Assistant Professor, I had continued my interest in the use of indomethacin for the treatment of premature labor. The ultrasound studies from my fellowship had taught us that the deleterious fetal effects of the drug could be monitored by a special type of ultrasound called a *fetal echocardiogram*. The Division of Pediatric Cardiology at the children's hospital was running short of internal research funding so I had agreed to pay part of the salary of a visiting research fellow from Italy. Dr. Moon was a dedicated researcher who had become quite proficient at performing fetal echos. Based on my previous research, the attending physicians were becoming more comfortable with the use of indomethacin for the treatment of premature labor in pregnancy. A fetal echo would need to be performed weekly in these patients to be sure that there were no ill effects on the fetus. I decided to have Dr. Moon perform the necessary echos. Because he was not a licensed physician, I would review the images and create a report. We would then bill the patient's insurance company for the indicated ultrasound. The monies would be placed in a special account to help pay for Dr. Moon's salary.

As such, the endeavor was no longer considered *research* but part of routine clinical care. Two years later, Dr. Moon left our university after being accepted as an OB-GYN resident at a northeastern ivy league school of medicine. Soon thereafter, I decided to have my research nurse pull all of the reports and the medical records of the patients to see if there was any differential effect of indomethacin on the fetus based on when the drug was used at different points in the pregnancy. I was also interested in seeing if the drug had different side effects in pregnancies with one fetus versus pregnancies with twins. My nurse reviewed all the records diligently and compiled a series of datasheets. For some reason, she decided to take these datasheets home one night but left them on the back seat of her car. The car was stolen that night. When found stripped of its wheels several days later by the police department, the datasheets were missing never to be seen again. My nurse was so upset over the incident that she decided to resign. A year later, I decided to resurrect the project from a list of patient names that I had retained on my office computer. All of the records were pulled a second time by my new research nurse. A statistician was paid to assist in the analysis of the data and a publication was later submitted to a major OB-GYN peer review journal with me as the sole author. The paper was accepted with minimal revisions and published shortly thereafter. Six months later, I received a call from Dr. Moon claiming that I had stolen his research data. He contested that he should have been an author on the paper since he had performed the echos. I pointed out that this series of patients was not considered research since we had billed the patients' insurance companies for the echo exams as part of clinical care (investigators are not allowed to bill patients for research studies that are not considered standard clinical care). Dr. Moon continued to protest. Later a conference call was arranged that included the OB-GYN Chairman of his department, my Chairman, Dr. Moon, and myself. At one point in the call, his Chairman requested that I submit the raw research data to him.

I responded, "Sir, with all due respect, you are not my boss. If you would like to register a complaint with the editors of the journal, I will be happy to comply with their requests for the data."

I never heard from the journal. Several years later, I was nominated for membership in a national research society. The chair from Dr. Moon's medical school objected to my nomination based on the authorship issue. My membership was tabled for one year until my new chair, Dr. Lo, could hear my story. After he defended me at the next annual meeting, I was allowed to enter the research society.

Allegations often haunt one's career for a long time. Years later when I was interviewing for the MFM Division Directorship at a mid-Atlantic medical school, I would have to recount my story again to contest the rumor that I "stole fellow research data."

15

A New Chair/New Financial Woes

Dr. Catch had served as Chairman of our OB-GYN department for the past twenty years (today's OB-GYN Chairman lasts on average six years). He realized that storm clouds were gathering for the impending financial crises that was soon to plague academic medical institutions. His goal was to continue his work at the microscope where he had become renowned as an expert in diseases of the female *vulva* (the skin that surrounds the outside of a woman's vagina). The medical school decided to call in a consultant to acquire some guidance as to the future direction of the department. After all, we were a *clinical* department, with several of the attendings being reported at the top of the list of highest earning academic physicians in the annual *U.S. News and World Report*. Dr. Lo was a well-known Chairman of OB-GYN at another institution and was considered one of the leading experts in the field of genetics. I met with him during a consulting visit to the department.

"We have a solid clinical practice here for patient care and resident training. What we need is more emphasis on academic productivity," I informed him.

One of the ploys of calling in a consultant is that it gives the person an opportunity to gather information on a program to see if they in fact may be interested in becoming a candidate for the lead position. In this case, the consultation request paid off. After several rounds of interviews and negotiations, Dr. Lo was named the new Chairman of our OB-GYN department. I once attended a leadership workshop sponsored by the *Association of Professors of OB-GYN*. A professor from the Wharton School of the University of Pennsylvania came to address us the first day.

"The way that you pick your leaders in academic medicine has always perplexed me," he said. "Let me make an analogy. The director of a welding shop decides it's time to retire. He looks around the shop and appoints his most skilled welder as the next director. What has just happened? The best welder is no longer working in the shop. More importantly this individual may be a great welder, but he may lack the skills to be a good leader."

After all, Dr. Lo was one of the most published OB-GYN academic physicians at that time. But how he would turn out as a leader of the department was yet to be determined.

Things got off to a rough start. Dr. Lo met with the group of senior MFM faculty who had developed lucrative private practices at the medical school. Dr. Catch, the former Chairman, had developed an incentive plan where the faculty kept 50% of patient billings after covering their individual expenses. The new Chairman proposed to put everyone on a fixed salary. This was not well received. Five of the MFM faculty decided to leave the department and create their own group private practice at a nearby hospital. Dr. Lo called me into his office.

"I have reviewed your academic accomplishments and I want to name you the new Director of the MFM Division."

"Have you talked with Dr. Winkle yet to let him know about the change?" I asked.

"I am going to give you that first tough task as a Division Director. I am going to let you chat with him," he replied.

In my mind, this did not seem to be the right way of doing things. After all Dr. Winkle had served in his role for more than twenty-five years. Was there no respect for the effort he had given to the medical school over all that time? I would soon learn over the coming years that this approach was not rare in academic medicine.

Even worse was my awkward position with my clinical mentor, Dr. Wood.

He had stopped by Dr. Lo's office to suggest: "I think Ken should run the inner-city hospital and I can run the private side of things. We can have a dual MFM Directorship."

"There will be one captain of the ship," I later was told was Dr. Lo's response. Wood decided to leave the department to set up his own private practice.

Part of the previous "fee agreement" that all the faculty had signed included a clause that allowed faculty to purchase capital equipment for their use using the 50% of their collections that they could not take home. This equipment was considered departmental property. Emotions were running high with the departure of the majority of the MFM Division. I had predicted that the faculty would not leave quietly. They would attempt to take as much equipment with them as possible. For this reason, I went to the private offices one evening and inventoried all of the ultrasound equipment. One day after the movers arrived, I noticed wires protruding from the walls where the ultrasound machines had been located. What remained of the Division faculty would therefore not have access to ultrasound equipment. Dr. Lo contacted the outgoing faculty. They were all asked to return the equipment based on their previous contractual agreements. They all acquiesced.

I had not yet talked with Dr. Winkle in my new position as Director of the Division. I wasn't sure how to break the news regarding the change in leadership. I received a phone call that made matters worse.

The head of the Hospital District administration that supervised the inner-city hospital called me. "Congratulations on your new appointment as Division Director. Well-deserved given all you have done for our patients during the two hospital moves. I need you to do something for me. I need you to address Dr. Winkle's alcohol use."

How many days had I been on this job? What else? I hesitated to go over and talk with Dr. Winkle. I went to his office at the hospital.

"Got a minute?" I asked.

"Sure," he said as he lit up another cigarette.

"There are a couple of things going on that I think you should know about since Dr. Lo's arrival," I said.

"Like what?" he responded.

"Well you know that I respect you immensely. I have been put in an awkward position. Dr. Lo has announced that I am the new Director of the MFM Division," I said. "I don't think this is the right way to do this. I think he should have talked to you first."

"Not surprising," he responded.

"Ok, I am glad we have that behind us. Then there is the issue that Ms. Mo wants me to talk to you about."

"And what is that?" he asked.

"Well she said we have to deal with your alcohol issue if you are to continue here in a position at the district." Dr. Winkle looked at me a little dismayed.

"Here is what I want to offer you. I may be speaking out of turn, but we will find the money to send you to a rehab facility out of state. The department will pay. I am not sure where I will find the money but that will be my problem," I said.

"Hmm, I would have to think that over," he replied.

"Mull it over a bit," I responded. "I will get back to you in a week or so."

The next week was busy. I spent most of the time trying to figure out how we were going to cover all the clinical services with only three other faculty and myself in a few short weeks. Dr. Winkle conspicuously avoided me. I finally ran into him a week later.

"Any thoughts yet on my proposal?" I asked.

"Not yet," he responded.

"Let me know when you are ready to chat," I replied. Another week went by—still no answer. Finally, two more weeks went by and I made an appointment to meet Dr. Winkle at this office.

"Well, we need to move forward on a decision," I proposed.

"I have given this a lot of thought my boy," he responded. "I am just not ready to do this. Appreciate the offer but this won't work for me."

I was dumbfounded. But then came one of the most difficult moments in my career.

"Well part of the plan was to have you stay over at the District. I have instructions from above that we have to ask you to retire if you will not accept this offer."

"Done," he responded.

I left the office wondering what I had gotten myself into in this new position. There was much more to come that I had yet to anticipate. I later was unable to attend Dr. Winkle's retirement party; it was scheduled late in the summer during my previously scheduled family vacation. I struggled with whether I should return in the middle of my vacation in order to attend the party but my wife made me commit to stay with the family. I learned that Dr. Winkle had a little too much to drink at his farewell event. He told everyone that I had prevented him from getting a job at a neighboring medical school. I knew better. They were aware of Dr. Winkle's long history of problems without my phone call.

When the new academic year rolled around, the mass exodus of MFM faculty left only three junior MFM faculty (all former fellows) and myself to cover a major inner-city obstetrical hospital, an outpatient private ultrasound unit, and a maternal transport service at the private hospital. The three current MFM fellows in training were asked to help out as well. All of us were taking in-house call every third night—shades of my past during residency. Dr. Lo, our new chair, and I had managed to recruit three new junior faculty but with the usual delay in getting hospital privileges, they would not be able to start until September first. It was a rough two months—I was exhausted.

With the new position as Chief of Obstetrics came new challenges—some more minor than others. I have had the opportunity to work with many different hospital administrators during the course of my career. Most of these folks that have an "O" in the initials that follow their job title (CEO, CFO, COO, CNO) usually work in a plush office on an upper floor of the hospital. They never enter the building the same way the patients do. They have a reserved parking place and come into the building through a rear entrance. They almost never leave their offices. Mr. Lard was not your typical hospital adminis-trator. At the reins of an inner-city hospital whose primary mission was to care for the indigent population of the city, he often faced significant challenges related to poor funding. Mike had the habit of making rounds on almost every floor of the building each morn-ing. He carried a set of pass keys and knew what was behind almost every door in the building. Often he would come by my office in the morning while he was making his rounds.

One of those visits was distinctly different. When he stuck his head in my door on that particular morning, I could see that his face was flushed.

"What's up?" I asked. I could tell he was visibly angry.

"Come with me," he instructed. The plans for our Labor and Delivery Unit had not included a *doctor's lounge*. The term is probably a misnomer. This room actually was a landing area for the OB-GYN residents and medical students. Although it did contain a television set, most of the activities in the room included working on medical charts or catching a few minutes of sleep between cases. Rarely was the television on. Nurses knew to go to the lounge if they need a resi-dent in the event of an emergency. Because a lounge had been forgot-ten in the planning of the Labor and Delivery Unit, a patient labor room had been pirated and converted. As we walked into the resident lounge, Mr. Lard pulled back the curtains to the outside window. The hinges on the frame had been noticeably altered to allow the window to swing wide open.

"Look at this!" he said as he pointed to the small roof area outside the window.

I peered outside. There strategically placed were several lounge chairs and a few standing ash trays. To say that this was a surprise finding for me would be an understatement. How many times had I been in this lounge and never peered past the window curtains. I felt like the father who just caught his daughter climbing out the window one night to rendezvous with her boyfriend. As I later investigated, the residents told me that the smokers in their group had reasoned this was a better alternative than going down to the emergency room to smoke in the designated area outside of the back door. Needless to say, I was instructed that the window would be fixed the next day by the hospital maintenance department. We were to dismantle the fire hazard area on the roof before then.

When there is a major change in leadership in an OB-GYN department, it was customary for the *ABOG* to undertake a site visit to be sure that the MFM fellowship is intact and that fellow training will be maintained. *ABOG* had hired a PhD educator to do the site visits. I had met Dr. Bird on several previous site visits. She was tough and to the point.

"No need for a ride from the airport. Only a tuna sandwich and a diet Coke for lunch," is all she ever asked for.

No frills. No way to be involved in an action that might present as an attempt to influence the outcome of her visit. Her biggest talent was being able to get the real facts as to what was really going on behind the scenes in a department. Were the fellows really being supervised or where they simply being abused as an extension of the faculty to see patients? I remember talking with her at her first visit to our fellowship when I was still in training.

During the interview she instructed me, "Everything that you are about to tell me is protected. Let's chat about what really goes on here."

Knowing that we had been in a tight spot for two months until our new junior MFM faculty began to see patients, I decided to meet with our current MFM fellows before the site visit.

"Now she is going to ask you to spill the beans behind closed doors. I want to let you know that we appreciate what you have done for the department these last two months. I do not want you to lie. I want you to remember all the things we were able to do together before these last two months."

I thought we would be fine. *ABOG* requires that there be a minimum of two board-certified MFM faculty in the Division to supervise the fellows to maintain the certification of the program. With the departure of so many faculty and the recruitment of only junior faculty, I was the only board-certified MFM remaining. I was able to recruit a mid-career MFM faculty from the other medical school in town who was board-certified. Surely with her letter of intent to join our Division, the board would see that we were going to continue to be a sound fellowship training program. I knew that our chair, Dr. Lo, was publicly critical of the MFM specialty in general. I figured this would not help our cause with *ABOG*. My biggest mistake was related to Dr. Fugue. In my preparation for the site visit, I had overlooked his special arrangement to join our training program from South Africa. He had completed two years of OB-GYN residency with us which we called his first and second year of residency training. During the next two years we treated him like an MFM fellow. Finally, after completing four years of "residency training," he was allowed to register with *ABOG* as an MFM fellow. In fact, Dr. Fugue functioned as an attending and was paid as such for the next two years. He was advanced enough in his research efforts that he was overseeing other MFM fellows in their research projects. But for Dr. Bird this was a glaring issue – a "fellow" overseeing the research thesis of another fellow. My bad! The letter from the board arrived about three weeks later—*ABOG* had put the fellowship on probation. The first real blow to my academic career. I was devastated. After my departure from the department a year later, the MFM fellowship would be officially closed two years later. It would not be reinstated at that institution for another decade.

Having coming from a state medical school, our Chairman was not used to a private medical school setting. At the monthly Division head meetings, we would review our budgets. They remained in the *red*. The large private hospital affiliated with our medical school did provide ongoing funds to balance our budget, but given that most of our obstetrical clinical activity was at the inner-city hospital or another competing private hospital, they were reluctant to continue to support the department. At the end of the first fiscal year, all the faculty were asked to take a 10% pay cut.

A year later, I was instructed to cut our faculty budget by an additional 20%. I met with each member of my Division and gave them one of two choices. We could all take a 20% pay cut and all five faculty that constituted the Division of MFM would retain their positions in the department or we could let go one faculty member go. I lobbied for the first choice at each of the individual meetings I held with the MFM faculty but the vote was unanimous—let one faculty member go. I announced the group's vote at the next MFM Division meeting. Everyone looked to their left and to their right.

Dr. Fugue spoke up. "Given all the crazy changes around here, I was thinking of leaving. I will start interviewing."

Two months later, he left to take a position in private practice in Utah.

Academic departments are more vulnerable to changes in the finances of health care than private practices. Medical schools in the past have placed more emphasis on teaching and research with clinical practice (and its associated revenues), ranking third on the list of priorities. For this reason, billing practices at academic practices are notoriously inefficient.

All medical procedures and patient visits are assigned a code—the *Current Procedural Terminology* or *CPT* code. This is a list of over 7,000 different codes that is maintained by the *American Medical Association*. When the bill for the physician's services is entered into the computer, it is linked to the *International Classification of Diseases (ICD)* code. This second code denotes the diagnosis of the patient's medical condition. In October 2015, the tenth edition of this coding went into effect in the USA, the *ICD-10* system. *ICD-10* is much more detailed than the older *ICD-9* system, with more than 69,000 codes as compared to the previous 14,000 codes. Some *ICD-10* codes seem a little superfluous such as the existence of a different code for the fracture of each bone of the finger (right and left hands have different codes). More outrageous are some of the new emergency medicine codes such as *V91.07XA—Burn due to water skis on fire*. Each *CPT* is assigned a composite numerical value for three different *Relative Value Units* or *RVU's*—an *RVU* value for physician work (52% of the effort), a value for practice expense (44%), and a value for professional liability insurance expense (9%). Currently Medicare reimburses at a rate of about thirty-two dollars for each *RVU* of the total *RVU's* for a procedure. Prior to the early 1990s, most payments for physician services were based on a *fee-for-service* basis. Fees varied widely across the country. Between 1986 and 1988, the U.S. Congress authorized a study to measure the work effort for more than 400 services performed by eighteen medical subspecialties. In early 1992, the U.S. Medicare program adopted a new payment system based on this *RVU* system. Today Medicaid and private insurers have also adopted this system.

But where has all the money gone, in medicine? I asked this question every day. Physicians are making approximately 30% less in salaries than fifteen years ago. Yet we spent $4.1 trillion on health care in the U.S. in 2021[56]. This equates to $12,318 each year for every man, woman, and child in our country. This is the highest expenditure per capita of any developed nation. I have asked many different individuals to weigh in on this to help decipher the answer. Although there are private hospital networks such as Hospital Corporation of America (HCA), many hospitals are awarded a *not-for-profit* status by local and federal governments. Because they are tax exempt, these hospitals are required to invest in resident education and to provide care for the underserved population. But all hospitals make a profit each year. In the 1980's, hospitals did exceptionally well and many invested their profits. Physicians also decided in some cases to build their own hospitals for subspecialty care such as orthopedics. Today, however, hospital budgets run on a slim margin. The industry has seen the closing of smaller hospitals, especially in rural areas. Acquisitions by larger hospital systems have resulted in many cities with only one or two competitive networks. The one outstanding exception to this trend has been the emergence of private emergency rooms. These facilities tout a shorter patient wait time than the usual hospital ER. However, in general they are associated with overutilization of imaging technology and higher overall costs. Recently, some major insurers have decided to withhold reimbursement for these services until a post-treatment review is undertaken on an individual patient's visit.

So what entities have profited from the increasing money spent in health care? Insurance companies are one answer. Insurance companies pay their administrators exceptionally high salaries, usually in the tens of millions of dollars annually. The CEO of Clover Health, a publicly traded heath insurance company, was paid $389 million in 2021[57]. The source of these funds is of course the premiums paid by the patient themselves or their employer on the patient's behalf. The *Affordable Care Act (ACA; also known as ObamaCare)* was passed in 2009, mandated that 80% of the premium dollars be spent by insurance companies on direct patient care or quality improvement projects[58]. Only 20% could be spent on administrative costs or marketing expenses. For insurance companies selling a policy to groups of more than fifty individuals, 85% of the premium dollar would have to be spent on patient care. In the past, executive salaries were deducted as a business expense in an effort to decrease federal taxes. The ACA limited these deductions to $500,000 and applied this to all executives of the insurance company. Another paradigm is the increasing reliance of state Medicaid programs on local Medicaid HMO companies. In Texas alone, as an example, there are more than twenty HMO's responsible for patient care. This allows each of these companies to use a percentage of the taxpayer dollar for administrative costs.

Finally one must look to the pharmaceutical and device industry for the sink hole of healthcare dollars in the USA. Early in my career, it was not uncommon for pharmaceutical representatives (*reps*) to sponsor lunches or dinners for the resident staff. This was done to "educate" them on the latest (and the most expensive) new medications. In OB-GYN offices, cabinets in outpatient clinics were "stocked" with samples of prenatal vitamins and oral contraceptives by these same reps. At some point, the pharmaceutical industry decided to shift its focus from marketing to physicians to direct patient advertising. I would love to have been in the boardroom when the marketing exec first proposed this paradigm switch. "Let's try selling our products to the patients instead of the doctors. They will go to their doctor's office and ask for our particular brand. We know physicians want to please their patients so they will write them the prescription for our drug." "Badda Book. Badda Boom" as they say on the Choice Hotels commercial. I am sure at least one board member objected. "This sounds crazy to me, but we will try it out on a limited basis." It is unlikely that particular board member still works for that company. One cannot watch television for more than a few minutes during the evening news to see direct patient advertising for everything from expensive monoclonal products for arthritis or psoriasis to "the purple pill" for *gastroesophageal reflux* (heartburn). I was especially overwhelmed one morning to see an advertisement on TV (these companies know the demographics of their audience and when to advertise certain products applicable to them) for a specific type of knee replacement device. "Ask your doctor for this superior device," the older patient was advised during the commercial. Can you imagine going to your trusted car mechanic and telling him, "I only want you to use brand X for my brake shoes when you do my brake job." Direct patient advertising is unique to the United States and New Zealand. Such advertising is outlawed in all other countries. Pharmaceutical companies (known as *pharma*) have a track record of paying handsome sums of money to physician leaders to consult or to be part of a speaker's bureau to provide lectures promoting their drugs. More recently, there has been a considerable backlash on these abusive practices. Many universities have enacted rules against pharma-sponsored lunches. Samples and pharma-labeled gifts such as computer mouse pads are banned from clinics. Physicians (and their immediate family members) are no longer allowed to hold stocks in companies where they serve as consultants. At each lecture and in conjunction with all scientific articles, any financial compensation from pharma must be disclosed.

But the real contribution of the pharmaceutical and device industry to the rising costs of health care can be attributed to the costs of the drugs and devices themselves. The United States leads the world in pharmaceutical development. The primary reason for this is the lucrative return on a successful product. *Research and development (R&D)* is expensive, and in our current regulatory environment, it can take ten to twelve years from drug discovery to market availability. This costs millions of dollars. New drug development begins with pre-clinical testing in both pregnant and non-pregnant animals to assess for toxic effects. The company must then submit an *Investigational New Drug (IND)* application for approval by the *Food and Drug Administration (FDA)* for a phase one clinical trial in normal human volunteers. This is allowed by a *phase two* trial in patients with the particular disease to determine the dose, side effects, and early efficacy. A *phase three* clinical trial follows at multiple research sites to determine the true effectiveness of the therapy. In this final phase of development, the drug is compared to a *placebo* (the equivalent of a sugar pill) in a *randomized study* (flip of the coin) to see if the claims of its benefits are real for a particular disease. Finally, all the data must be submitted to the *FDA* with a check for one million dollars before the product can be marketed. *Phase four* involves collecting information on unexpected side effects once the drug is being used by the general population. All drug development is a risk. The early exciting benefits seen in animal models may not be realized in human subjects. Even worse, significant side effects may cause the *FDA* to stop a drug from going to market or the drug may be removed from the market after it receives *FDA* approval due to unanticipated side effects in a large population. I once asked a pharma CEO how they priced a particular drug once the company's R&D had been recovered from the early sales of the drug.

"Do you decrease the costs of the drug at that point ?" I asked.

"Nope," he replied. "We are like an oil and gas company. We drill a hole where our geologist tells us there should be oil. Many times, we end up with a dry hole and we have lost all the costs in drilling that well. Every now and then we hit a gusher. We use that money to drill the next hole."

Although this makes sense at face value, there is still the reality of the astronomical charges for medications that are newly approved by the FDA. Take a new gene therapy recently approved by the FDA to treat spinal muscular atrophy—an inherited disease that in its most common form results in 82% of affected children dying by age four. Approximately 6,000 affected children are born in the U.S. annually. Novartis, the drug's manufacturer, set the initial charge for the drug at $2.1 million; however, they are willing to allow insurance companies to pay out the costs over five years at $425,000 annually. I calculated that if all 6,000 babies received the drug—the total costs to the U.S. healthcare system would be over $2.1 billion! I am not the one to question the need for such a life-saving therapy, nor is society as a whole ready to say this is too expensive to provide this to these patients. Yet are these types of costs sustainable in the future for all the other innovative discoveries yet to be conceived? Recently there have been discussions at the federal governmental level to enact legislation to have pharma delineate the cost of drugs at the time of their advertisement. Currently most companies simply state that there are ways to apply for reduced costs if your insurance carrier does not pay for the drug. Pharma has pushed back on this legislation. They have proposed to simply provide a website (the http address might be found at the bottom of the television screen in fine print) where the consumer can be directed to get pricing. My guess is that their intent is to minimize the chance for real transparency.

The second academic year with our new Chairman began.

On July 15, my wife called me. "Have you seen your paycheck this month? You received a 20% pay cut."

"Can't be," I responded. "We balanced our Divisional budget with Dr. Fugue's leaving. There was no discussion of a pay cut for me."

"Well I compared it to last year's check and it is definitely there," she responded.

I called Dr. Lo's office. His secretary answered.

"I need to meet with Dr. Lo right away," I said.

"He is a bit tied up all day today. Can you meet with him tomorrow?" she responded.

"No, this is important, I need to meet with him today," I said.

"I just don't think that will be possible," she replied.

"Well I am headed over to sit on the couch outside of his office. When he takes a bathroom break, I'll follow him and we can discuss the change in my paycheck," I said. Dr. Lo met with me an hour later.

"I noticed that my check this month includes a 20% reduction. What gives?" I asked.

"Well, Ken we talked about this already. You had to do this to balance the budget."

"No sir," I responded. "I did what you asked me to do. I balanced the Division's clinical budget. A pay cut was not what I expected. I will tell you how I know this. When you handed out a 10% pay cut last year, I made a promise to my wife that if I received a second pay cut this year, I would leave and find another job. Here I sit here in front of you, so I know we have not discussed this second pay cut. I have lost total trust in you."

"What will I have to do to win back your trust?" he asked.

"I am not sure that's possible," I replied. The next day, I began to look for new opportunities for my academic career.

In the course of an academic career, an attending physician on average will change institutions three or four times. My career was no exception. I had expected to retire at my first medical school appointment. After all I had spent thirteen years at the program, had been promoted from a fellow to a tenured full professor, and had been selected to head the MFM Division and fellowship training program. Salaries at medical schools do not mirror those in corporate America. In my almost forty years in academic medicine, I remember receiving only one cost of living raise and one actual raise. True there has been the occasional bonus at the end of the fiscal year if the Division did better than expected for its projected budget. All of the other increases in my salary were negotiated at the time of recruitment to a new medical school position. The reason for these static salaries is simple—few academic physicians understand where the money comes from. Most think that because they have the privilege to be appointed to a medical school, big brother should take care of them. In the next phase of my academic career, this issue was about to hit me square in the face.

16

East Coast Brings New Challenges: The Electronic Medical Record and the Death of Colleagues

My wife was from a mid-Atlantic state on the East Coast. She had followed a medical student who was starting a surgical residency at the same institution where I started my OB-GYN residency. She was a Labor and Delivery nurse so we both started work on the same day that I started by OB-GYN internship at the university hospital. We became good friends through our discussions over cups of coffee during late night shifts. Eventually she would become engaged to her medical student. I was distraught! Two months later, the engagement was off. We began dating in the spring of my intern year. We were married three years later. Soon after my salary discussion with Dr. Lo, I learned of an open MFM Division Director position at a prestigious *little ivy* medical school on the East Coast. This presented an opportunity to move Karen and our three girls back with her family.

An interview trip was arranged and I met with most of the members of the MFM Division during my visit. One of the things that attracted me to the position was their new chair—Dr. Papel. She was an impressive individual. At a time when most of the leadership positions in our specialty were dominated by male figures, Dr. Papel had risen through the ranks to become the president of our national MFM organization, a key member of *ABOG*, and was assuming her second Chairmanship of a major OB-GYN department. I had previously worked with her in my position as fellowship Director at my first institution. At that time, she was the MFM Division Director and Director of the MFM fellowship at the neighboring medical school. I had tremendous respect for her. We met a month after my interview trip at our national MFM society meeting. I had only one reservation about working for her.

"I have talked with some of my colleagues. They tell me that when the chair is in the same specialty as the Division Director, there can be major differences of opinion on clinical programs. Would you be comfortable if I ask you to take off your chair hat every now and then to allow me to address you not as my boss, but as a member of my Division?" I asked.

"Works for me," she said.

Over the next hour we discussed issues like salaries, endowed professorships, and a wish list for the needs of the Division. I watched as she took notes on her clean white linen napkin from the restaurant. When we were finished talking, she pushed the napkin across the table to me.

"Take a look at this and see what we need to change," she said.

I crossed out the salary figure and penned a higher number. I pushed it back across the table. Other items went back and forth a few times on the napkin. We then agreed we liked the final list on the napkin. Dr. Papel put the white piece of linen in her purse as we left the restaurant. Two days later I received a formal written offer letter. I signed and dated it the same day. I would use the *napkin* method in several future recruitments as a MFM Division Director.

I walked into the MFM office suite at my new university on July first. Things were eerily quiet. I found the lead secretary for the Division sitting at a desk full of papers in the main area of the suite.

"Where are all the faculty?" I asked.

"They're all on vacation," she responded. The faculty take their vacations during the summer when the main campus of the university is out for summer break."

"Well, who is taking care of the patients?" I asked.

"The fellows," she replied. I knew at once that many challenges would lie ahead.

Several days later, I took my first night of call on Labor and Delivery. One of the private attending patients of the MFM Division was laboring when I arrived for my night shift. At about 3 a.m., I was preparing for the vaginal delivery of her baby.

"Can I get a delivery tray?" I asked the patient's nurse. I was immediately handed a small blue plastic tray about the size of a cigar box. I pulled the seal off the top. In the tub were two small gauze, an umbilical cord clamp and a hemostat.

"Can I ask what this is?" I asked.

"It's the *home delivery* tray," she proudly announced.

"But we stopped doing home deliveries in the late 1900s in this country; aren't we in a hospital?" I asked.

The next day I called the scrub nurses at the inner-city hospital at my old institution. "I am in desperate need of a list of instruments on the delivery tables. Can you please send me this list?" I asked. Two weeks later we had a complete set of instruments for all deliveries. Dr. Papel, the chairperson, took in-house call on Friday nights to maintain her clinical skills. After her first night of call after my arrival, she came by my office.

"I have a list of issues that need to be addressed on the unit. Can you start to whittle away at these?" she asked.

This time she did not produce a napkin. Instead she pulled out a long piece of toilet paper from her scrubs. Scribbled in ink on about ten squares was a list of various items. Five or six call nights later, the list from the chair became more abbreviated and was written on only two toilet paper squares. Several months later, I knew I was making progress when I received only an email with two items after the chair had taken her night of call.

Although I have always favored *walk rounds* with the residents, the tradition at this particular institution was for all of the MFM attendings to participate in a *morning report* format with the senior residents on the service. The nurses were notably excluded. Afternoon check out rounds for the residents that would be covering the OB service at night took place in a small room behind the central nurses' station in Labor and Delivery. There was a small window between the two areas. The routine practice was for the attending to lower the blinds at the window to exclude the nurses from listening in.

On one particular morning soon after I arrived, a patient was presented at morning report with a suspected *placenta previa*. In this situation the patient's placenta is implanted low in the uterus and can cover the cervix. This complicates only 1%–2% of pregnancies. Should labor contractions begin, catastrophic bleeding can occur. As a result, these patients are routinely delivered by C-section. After the presentation, a senior faculty member recommended the patient be taken back for a *double set-up*. Now, I had only read about doing this in older obstetrical textbooks. In this scenario, the patient is brought to the operating room and preparations are made for a C-section. The OB does a vaginal examination to see "if they feel the placenta" through the cervix. This has the potential to induce significant bleeding. If bleeding starts or the placenta is palpated, a C-section is undertaken. The practice at my original institution had moved well beyond this. Ultrasound could be undertaken with a special probe that is placed in the vagina and one can see exactly where the placenta is located without any risk of bleeding. The senior attending at my new institution trained in the pre-ultrasound era and was unaware of the newer modality to safely diagnose a *placenta previa*.

This case illustrates an important aspect of academic medicine. In our political system, there are term limits. When a new administration comes in, there is a total change of personnel. This has the advantage of a fresh start and a new perspective. The downside is that often there is no *corporate memory*. There are no *term limits* in academic medicine. Tenured professors may stay at one institution for many years. In addition, many academic divisions are built by retention of trainees from the institution's fellowship program. Fellows are trained in the practice patterns of their senior attendings. The better ones are retained as junior faculty at the conclusion of their training. This leads to tremendous *in-breeding* with poor acceptance of new innovative ideas. I was the outsider at this new institution. I was clearly perceived as the *maverick*. Change would be difficult to implement. Dr. Papel and I would later brainstorm about what individuals liked *change*. We decided it was limited to babies with dirty diapers, panhandlers, and prisoners.

It was my birthday at the end of my first month of my new Directorship. I was the attending on the OB service that day. A patient had been taken back for a C-section and a partial *placenta accreta* had been unexpectantly discovered. *Placenta accreta* is a one of the most feared complications of obstetrics. In most cases of normal implantation of the placenta on the uterine wall, the placenta is easily removed at the time of delivery with a simple tug on the umbilical cord or a swipe of the hand at the time of C-section. In the case of *placenta accreta*, the placenta implants over an old scar on the womb (many times the one left over from a previous C-section). It then grows into the muscle of the uterus. Attempts at removal result in major bleeding and the need for a hysterectomy. When I arrived in the operating room, attempts at removing the placenta had already resulted in major blood loss for the patient. We proceeded with a hysterectomy, but by then the patient had lost so much blood that her normal mechanism for forming blood clots was compromised. So, we placed several gauze packs on the raw surgical surfaces and allowed our anesthesiologist to administer the correct blood products to fix the clotting problem. After about thirty minutes, we removed the packs and the bleeding had stopped. In every surgery, the scrub technician who is handing instruments to the surgeons has the primary responsibility of counting all instruments and gauze pads. This is done before the surgery is started and then done twice at the end of the case. This is to assure that one of the cardinal mistakes of surgery does not occur—a retained sponge or instrument. I asked the scrub tech in our case to confirm that the initial sponge and instrument count was correct. She confirmed it was.

I then asked the senior resident, "You OK closing?".

"Sure," was the response.

I left the operating room to dictate the operative note into the medical record. The final count after closure of the skin was correct as well. Two days after the surgery, the patient developed a fever and was placed on antibiotics. Due to a somewhat poor response, a CT scan was ordered which demonstrated an *abscess* (a localized collection of infected material) in the lower part of the patient's abdomen. After a week of antibiotics, the fever subsided and the patient went home. The patient did develop some problems with an infection in her C-section skin incision but she was managed in the clinic as an outpatient. In late August, she presented to our emergency room with increasing drainage from her C-section incision. A CT scan was ordered.

The MFM fellow called me at home that night, "You might want to come in and see this patient."

I arrived at the hospital to look at the films with him. There were two retained lap sponges in the area of the previous *abscess*. When then reviewed the first CT scan. Although the majority of the CT images were suggestive of an *abscess*, the *scout film* (a little picture that shows the level of all the cross-sectional images of the CT scan that appears on the bottom right on the main film) clearly showed the lap sponges. Because cotton gauze, like metal surgical instruments, does not show up on X-rays, all gauze items have a metallic dye impregnated in them to allow them to be detected. On the *scout film*, the two metallic stripes could be easily appreciated. How could two lap sponges be missed on the two final surgical counts? And we were not off by one sponge, but two! The patient was taken back to surgery the next day and the sponges were removed. After she filed a lawsuit, the radiologist admitted at his deposition that he rarely looks at the *scout film* and the cross-sections of the CT scan still looked to him like it demonstrated an *abscess*. At my deposition, I could only tell the plaintiff's attorney that I felt that we had removed all the sponges based on the scrub tech's first count. As the *captain of the ship* for the case, I had to assume the ultimate responsibility for the error. The patient decided to *settle* the case for the price of a particular used car she always wanted. The hospital waived all of her remaining medical expenses. I decided we needed to modify our current hospital practice. Previously, sponges were placed on the floor to be counted. All sponges would now have to be placed in a special counting bag that was placed on a vertical pole for easy visualization—one sponge per bag. Subsequently, I was also known to hide an occasional sponge between my hip and the surgical table to see if the final count would be correct. To my knowledge, no other cases of retained sponges at a C-section occurred on our OB service for the next eight years of my tenure.

A few years after this initial incident, two lawsuits were brought against the obstetrical service for retained gauze sponges left in the vagina at the time of routine Ob deliveries. The patients presented several weeks after going home with a foul-smelling vaginal discharge. One patient even claimed that she had developed an infection in her tubes that was going to impact her future fertility. An investigation revealed that the OB-GYN residents had placed a four-inch by four-inch gauze pad in the vagina when they were suturing a vaginal laceration after a delivery. This kept any bleeding coming from the uterus from obstructing their view. Then they would forget and leave the gauze in place. I had been taught during my residency training to perform a "digital sweep" of the vagina as the last maneuver after completing a vaginal delivery. This was a preventative move that allowed one to detect any gauze that might have been left in the vagina at the conclusion of the procedure. Although this seemed simple enough, our QA committee met and decided a better preventative maneuver was to replace the smaller gauze sponges with a longer lap sponge. With the larger gauze, a portion would have to remain outside of the vagina at all times. Thereafter, retained sponges after vaginal delivery no longer presented a problem.

A few weeks later, my wife was sitting on the bleachers watching my daughter's softball game. She struck up a conversation with another mom sitting next to her. "Where do you work?" my wife asked.

"I am a nurse at the university hospital," she responded.

"What's it like to work there?" my wife asked.

"Well it was fine until recently. Then this new faculty came in and everything is changing."

"Would his name be Dr. Moise?" my wife inquired.

"How did you know that?" she replied.

"I am married to him." The conversation went silent at that point. Both women turned their attention to the softball game.

One of my next big projects was to introduce an electronic record or EMR to the obstetrical service. Just before I left my previous institution, I had been approached by an Israeli software firm that was developing a *smart* electronic chart. The group was interested in partnering with an academic medical center to help develop the rules engine for the chart that would remind the user when they were not following nationally accepted clinical guidelines for acceptable OB care. I knew at the time that I was leaving for my new institution but was able to convince the Israeli group to work with me in my new position. A few months after my arrival, I began to hold a series of workshops with the MFM faculty to design acceptable reminders for clinicians when they missed certain aspects of the pregnant patient's care. After about six months of work, we were ready to implement. Training sessions were held with both the nursing and physician staff.

We felt we had anticipated every problem. We were soon to realize otherwise. The day we went live with the chart, an obstetrical patient presented in labor with twins with complete cervical dilation—delivery was eminent. There was no time to even get the patient a medical record number to be able to open the EMR. This required us to modify the software to allow for a *Jane Doe* feature for similar future situations. A new record could be opened and the patient identifications added when there was time after the acute clinical scenario had calmed. The EMR software had been written so that both the nurses' and physicians' progress notes were displayed on the same screen. Given the culture at the institution, physicians found this to be unacceptable.

"Why would they need to see the nurses' notes?" they asked.

To address this issue, another major modification to the software was undertaken—progress notes could be displayed after filtering to an "all" view or only a physician or nursing view could be selected. This seemed to satisfy the general reluctance of the healthcare workers to continue to implement the EMR. Clinical reminders appeared on the computer screen based on previously agreed upon rules. This too proved problematic. The faculty thought the reminders were excessive and again they wanted them to be filtered to only those appropriate for the physicians and those appropriate for the nurses to be displayed. A situation then arose where a nurse had taken an initial history from a patient who stated she was allergic to codeine. The patient stated that she developed nausea—a common *side-effect* of codeine that does warrant a designation of an allergy. The nurse entered an allergy to codeine in the EMR. The resident physician then talked with the patient and determined that the reaction to codeine was indeed a side effect and not a true allergy. She overwrote the allergy that the nurse had entered and changed the allergy field to "none". This caused a major disruption between the nurses and the physicians. I pointed out that the EMR kept an electronic log of all alterations to the chart as well as the identification of the provider that made the alteration. This did not appease the nurses—whose license would be on the line if the nurse went on to give codeine and the patient had a major life-threatening complication. Who would take the blame? Several of the senior OB nurses threatened to resign over this situation. As a result, the Director of nursing convinced the hospital administration that the EMR project was a failure and that the effort should be discontinued. Clearly the nurse/physician culture at the time did not allow for such a progressive experiment— we were too far ahead of the curve. The EMR would not be universally introduced into medicine for another five years.

One of the biggest changes in health care has been the implementation of the EMR. At the turn of the century, American physicians documented the progress of their patients in a written diary. The goal was to create a record of experiences that could be used for teaching and sharing information with other colleagues. Later the American College of Surgeons prompted the use of a written record for hospitalized patients.

For many decades, patients' medical records were recorded on paper. At the time of their admission to the hospital, a physician would have to request the patient's previous chart (usually located in a medical records storage area in the basement of the hospital) to review past hospital admissions. The medical chart for the patient's current admission was often kept in a metal or plastic binder in the *chart rack* located at the nursing station on each floor. Daily physician notes regarding the patient's hospital course (known as *progress notes*) were handwritten and many times difficult to read based on the legibility of the physician's penmanship. The initial history and physical after the patient was first admitted, operative notes, and the final discharge summary were often dictated into a transcription system and appeared in the medical record as a typed note a day or so later. This practice greatly enhanced clarity. The first introduction of electronic systems in hospitals was to retrieve laboratory results and X-ray reports.

Although computers and the internet have improved the quality of our lives and made once difficult to find services easy to locate with the simple click of a mouse, the EMR has not proven to be as beneficial to healthcare as once proposed. In 2009, the federal legislation known as the *American Recovery and Reimbursement Act* was passed to prevent a major economic recession after several major banks became insolvent due to subprime home mortgages. Part of this stimulus package included twenty-seven billion dollars in incentive payments to physicians and their practices caring for *Medicare* and *Medicaid* patients to promote implementation of an EMR[59]. *The Affordable Care Act* passed one year later had additional language that endorsed the use of the EMR. There were several problems with this effort to stimulate the implementation of the EMR. The first major shortfall was that the legislation did not include the need for a common format or language so that the various software products could easily talk to one another. In contrast, *interoperability* was realized as a need in the early phase of computerization of the banking industry. As a result, one can use an ATM card at one bank automated teller and obtain funds from a different bank where one's funds are kept. The lack of cross-talk between EMRs has become even more problematic as different software vendors were chosen by each hospital system. The second major problem with the EMR implementation was that the vendors programmed the software to optimize billing opportunities and not for ease of documentation by healthcare workers. The federal financial incentives were therefore the major driver for software development. Extensive physician training sessions were required for implementation. Hospitals and clinics were told to reduce their patient census by 50% during the early phases of implementation. *The MD Anderson Cancer Center* experienced such a reduction in revenue during the period when they implemented an EMR that they decided to downsize "non-essential" personnel by over 1,000. With the paper chart, nurses and physicians routinely used written *free text* to describe their interactions with their patients. Even operative notes were not standardized—the physician could dictate the procedure with his own style of narration. In an outpatient setting, I could carry a hand-held recording device and dictate notes between seeing patients as I walked from exam room to exam room. My secretary would then type these and they would appear in the chart twenty-four hours later. Computerized records are much more restrictive. Written using database software, free text opportunities are more limited and boxes have to be checked with drop-down menus for many fields. If one does want to free text a comment, it has to be typed. When I was being taught by the Jesuits in high school, my classmates and I asked if we could take some form of a typing class. In the typical paternalistic nature of the Jesuits, we were informed "you will always have a secretary. We need to teach you things like Latin, not typing." The Jesuits clearly did not have the vision that computers would someday change our lives. Children in elementary school today are no longer taught script handwriting; instead, they are taught to type on computers. Although millennials are used to interacting with computers by using a keyboard for the EMR, they have also learned to game the system by using the *cut and paste* option. Previous notes are used as a template for notes entered on a later encounter in the patient's chart. Even more problematic is the use of notes from other patients' charts that are pasted into a new patient's record. Without careful proofing, these *cut and paste* options lead to countless errors. Baby boomers like myself have to learn new typing skills that far exceed their previous "hunt and peck" approach. Voice recognition software is improving; however, the products for medical dictation remain somewhat limited. Due to its cumbersome structure, the EMR has actually decreased physician efficiency. A recent study found that female primary care physicians actually do a better job documenting in the EMR by spending 19% more time than their male counterparts[60]. Unfortunately, this puts them at an unfair advantage in a *value-based payment model* where their salary is based on the total number of patient visits. It also increases their *pajama time*—a new term that has emerged to describe the time spent at home completing a physician's medical records from patients seen that day.

Two of the current EMR products, Epic® and Cerner®, now account for more than 56% of market share[61]. Yet when judged on usability by health providers, Epic® ranks number two and Cerner® ranks number six[62]. The lack of usability has led to additional personnel hires in some venues. In busy outpatient clinics or emergency rooms, *scribes* are hired to contemporaneously enter data into the EMR while the physician examines a patient or takes their history. In some institutions, outsourcing to countries like India has been the answer. Unemployed physicians in India are employed as *scribes* to enter data into the EMR as they listen to a U.S. physician perform a physician examination while dictating the results.

Hardware issues also contribute to the problems with ease of use of the EMR. Hospitals did not invest in mobile computer tablets but decided to add PCs at nursing stations or occasionally to mount them on the wall of a ward. Later *COWS* appeared ("computers on wheels" with a battery attached). Clearly this was the hospital's cost savings answer as opposed to putting PCs in all of the patient rooms. The EMR has created new personnel costs to the medical system. A platoon of information technology support personnel must be available around the clock to support the software and hardware. A twenty-four hour help desk must be maintained to assist physicians with password updates.

This lack of insight on the limitations of the hardware has resulted in a significant impact on the physician / patient interaction as well. With paper charts, the physician would face the patient and scribble a few notes while interacting directly with the patient during a clinic visit. This allowed them to spend the entire time talking and examining the patient. Now the physician must face a computer screen on the wall and type in their notes. In summary the EMR has dehumanized the patient.

A recent survey of 15,000 physicians from twenty-nine specialties indicated that the percentage of physicians reporting burnout was lowest in public health (29%), while urology ranked near the top (54%)[63]. Use of an EMR was felt to be a contributing factor. For every one hour of patient interaction, providers reported the need for an additional two hours for computer-based documentation and order entry[64]. Male physicians are more than 1.4 times more likely to undertaken suicide when compared to the general male population while female physicians are more than 2.3 times as likely than their general population counterparts.

One would think that a *smart* EMR could be developed to reduce medical errors. This has yet to happen. A *smart* EMR might include reminders that would appear on the screen when a health provider forgets to order a lab test or fails to check a result. The current generation of EMRs lacks these reminders. In fact, the EMR may actually lead to an increase in medical errors. In Samuel Shen's latest book, *Man's 4th Best Hospital*, the "fat man" from the *The House of God* returns to unite his former intern class to develop a utopian clinic[65]. He points out, "The EMR is like texting while driving—the cause of many mistakes."

When a paper chart was used, all Rh-negative women who were pregnant had their charts stamped with a red text "RH NEGATIVE."

It was virtually impossible to miss the injection of Rhesus immune globulin that is the *standard of care* to administer at 28 weeks gestation. Without this injection, about one in 100 women will develop antibodies that may harm their offspring in their future pregnancies. And once this occurs, there is no reversing the process. All future pregnancies have the chance to be affected. I recently reviewed several medical records to render an expert opinion in cases of missed Rhesus immune globulin.

I asked the attorney, "Why do you think these cases are happening?"

"Easy," she replied. "It's the EMR. The nurse and the physicians have to scroll through multiple screens to see the patient's blood type. It's just not right there in front of them like it was on the old paper record."

Reading information on a computer screen in itself may contribute to some of these errors. A recent study of seventy-two volunteers at a Swedish university was conducted to assess their scores on a standardized reading comprehension entrance examination[66]. Subjects read five 1,000-word passages and then answered multiple-choice questions. Scores were significantly lower when the tests were taken on the computer as compared to the subject taking the test on paper. Another study by the same group looked at taking the exam on the computer by scrolling the screens as compared to having the information displayed one page at a time. Subjects were then asked to perform a series of cognitive tests. Those who were administered the entrance exam with scrolling performed more poorly on the post-exam cognitive testing. In another study in Norway, tenth-graders given a reading comprehensive test on paper as compared to reading it on a computer scored lower on their exams when the computer was used.

One day I found myself on a plane flight headed to a medical meeting. Now usually I bring academic work along with me so I am often not that sociable with the fellow travelers sitting next to me. This day was uniquely different—I had caught up with most of my work. The passenger in the seat next to me introduced himself, "Hi, I am Dave."

"Ken here," I replied. "What do you do for a living?" I asked.

"I am a computer programmer for an EMR software company," he replied.

"Wow, I am one of those physicians that has to use your EMR," I replied. What an opportunity to share my frustration with EMRs to one of the very individuals who created one!

After about twenty minutes of conversation, he asked me, "So why don't physicians want to use EMRs?"

I carefully thought about my choice of words so as to not offend him. After a few moments, I reached into my pocket and pulled out a pen.

"See this pen," I said. "It is constantly with me. I don't have to find it. It never runs out of power. And best of all, it gives me total freedom to say what I want about a patient. When your EMR can match all that, then all of us will be onboard."

Despite the general frustration with the EMR, it is here to stay. Clearly the issue of enhanced usability needs to be addressed in version 2.0. Perhaps we can use voice recognition and natural language processing to capture important data points. Perhaps an intelligent chart can help us with diagnoses and help us reduce human errors.

A senior mentor once told me "Don't leave a job just because you are unhappy. Leave because you are going to a better place. All jobs have their hidden problems."

That was sound advice. One of the attractions of accepting the position at the East Coast medical school was its junior MFM faculty. I had met Dr. McKiney during my interview process. He had just finished the MFM fellowship at the same medical school and had stayed on faculty as an Assistant Professor. While he was in the fellowship, he was motivated enough to complete his Masters in Public Health degree at the same time. Dr. McKiney had already published a paper in the prestigious *New England Journal of Medicine*. We had lunch together when I saw him at our MFM society's national meeting in February before I had accepted the position of MFM Director at his institution.

"Where are all the research papers from your department?" I asked.

"Not something emphasized in our Division," he replied.

"Well where are all the MFM fellows?" I inquired again.

"They have to stay home so all the faculty can come to the meeting."

"What do you think about that?" I asked.

"I don't think that is the way it should be, but that's the current culture," he replied.

Clearly he and I were on the same page of the need for a culture shift if I accepted the position as the new head of MFM at his department.

Dr. McKiney was a big runner. He was training to run in the Boston marathon later that year. In August, one month after I arrived in my new position, I received a call from him.

He was crying on the phone. "I just couldn't get my training schedule to advance so I went in to have a blood test to check for anemia. My white blood cell count was 80,000 (normal is 6—10,000). They think I may have leukemia. I am being admitted in a few hours to have a bone marrow biopsy. I thought you should know."

"No problem, your health is most important. Don't worry about your clinical assignments."

The next day the bone marrow biopsy showed acute myeloid leukemia. This is a terrible disease in young adults. At that time the five-year survival for Dr. McKiney's age group was 58% with the best of new therapies[67]. Dr. McKiney was admitted to the oncology service and underwent intensive chemotherapy. It was later determined that one of his brothers was an excellent "match" so he underwent a bone marrow transplant. Nine months elapsed. Dr. Papel and I decided to keep him on full salary. I made arrangements to have his office computer moved to his hospital room so he could continue to work on research projects when he felt up to it. After about a year, he met with me and asked if he could re-enter clinical care.

"Let's take it slow," I said. No call or daytime Labor and Delivery coverage. We'll just put you seeing patients in the clinic a couple of days a week," I replied.

Later McKiney offered to give grand rounds for the Department of OB-GYN. He would tell his story as a patient with the perspective of a physician. In my thirty-year career, I can remember perhaps a handful of lectures that made a deep impression on me. McKiney's grand rounds was one of these. He began with a humorous story where the hematologist arrived to perform his first bone marrow biopsy. Upon opening the instrument tray, he remembers the attending getting a perplexed look.

"What is this?" the attending had asked. McKiney had glanced over—it was a circumcision tray.

"Won't need that today," he admonished. "Already had that done some years ago".

Seems that the circumcision tray and the bone marrow instrument tray order numbers were only one digit different. McKiney recounted the bad times as well. While experiencing extreme nausea from chemotherapy, he was scheduled to be taken to radiology for X-rays. The orderly arrived pushing the transport stretcher eating a jelly donut. Just the sight of this brought on additional waves of nausea. There was not a dry eye in the audience as he concluded his talk with a description of his worse days.

"Did you know that when you get intensive chemotherapy, you slough the calluses from the soles of your feet? This becomes so painful that when you finally get a shower you can feel every grout line of the tile on the floor of the shower."

At one of our MFM Division meetings that McKiney was able to attend, I was presenting the annual budget. We were close to the line with revenue and expenses but we would be OK for the next fiscal year. There would be no bonuses.

Dr. Cole, a professed "friend" of McKiney spoke, "Why then are we paying sick people a full salary?" he asked.

There was complete silence in the room. I must admit it took me a good fifteen seconds to process a response.

"Dr. Papel and I talked about this and felt that because McKiney is participating in ongoing research efforts, this was fair. Should any other member of the Division become sick, we would treat them the same way," I responded.

Three weeks later I received an urgent phone call from the hospital patient relations department. McKiney had experienced a grand mal seizure while examining a patient in the clinic. The patient had complained to the hospital. The clinic nurses had failed to mention anything to me. I knew this was not a good sign. Recurrent AML can present with metastasis to the brain. McKiney knew it too, yet he decided to forego any imaging studies. A month later, he was volunteering at a summer children's camp for oncology survivors when he was found disoriented in the woods. The MRI the next day showed multiple areas of metastasis in his brain. His oncologist offered to treat him with whole brain radiation—not curative but it could prevent further seizures. I did what I knew he would do if he had felt better—search the medical literature to understand the pros and cons of the therapy. The data did not look good. Changes in personality and cognition were not unusual after whole brain irradiation. I shared this with him. McKinney decided to have the therapy anyway. Afterwards his treating physicians decided to try a repeat bone marrow transplant with his brother again serving as the donor. This time *graft-vs-host disease* (the donor bone marrow cells actually begin to kill off the patient) occurred and it appeared that all further therapeutic attempts would be futile. I met with McKinney to get permission to talk with this oncologist. I offered to move him to long-term disability insurance which by university standards was very generous paying three quarters of his salary. McKinney was single. During his two-year ordeal his mother had moved to our town to care for him. She never left his side. In the last months she took care of him at his home until he finally passed away. I grieved a great loss of a gifted individual.

In the past, denial of coverage by private health insurance companies for pre-existing medical conditions and caps on total medical care were commonplace. When the *Affordable Care Act* passed in 2010, insurance restrictions on both of these parameters were forbidden[68]. By the time he had completed both of his bone marrow transplants, McKiney's medical expenses had approached $900,000. The insurance cap for our university health plan at the time was one million dollars. Had he lived longer, McKiney would have had to forego his salary and apply for Medicaid assistance.

I would have to face death once again during the eight short years I was at the mid-Atlantic university. Bob was a middle-aged PhD I had hired to run my rabbit lab. When I was back at my original medical school department, I had managed to find local grant funding to develop an animal model for *hemolytic disease of the fetus and newborn (HDFN)*. The only real therapy for this disease was intrauterine transfusion—placing a needle into the fetus or its umbilical cord to give it red blood cells. But this procedure could result in complications and even fetal loss. We needed something better. Rabbits had been used back in the 1950s to study red blood cell problems in pregnancy. Working with an immunologist, I had re-created a rabbit *HDFN* model but increased the complexity by introducing ultrasound and blood sampling of the fetuses[69]. When I left for my new job, we had to ship all forty rabbits in the colony to their new home on the East Coast. It was not an easy trip for them. Born in an air-conditioned room, they had never seen sunshine or experienced heat. Sitting in their cages on the loading dock at 3 a.m., they lay there panting in the heat. Once in the air-conditioned transport vehicle, they were home free.

Bob was a unique individual. He had previously worked as a photographer for *National Geographic* magazine and had traveled all over the world in that capacity. I charged him with continuing the work with the rabbits that I had started to develop so that intrauterine transfusions would not be needed in the HDFN-affected pregnancies.

We were in the lab working together one day when I noticed some extensive scarring on Bob's legs.

"If you don't mind me asking, were you in a car accident in the past?" I asked.

Our university maintained a small airport in the town. Although used primarily for university business, a small flying club was based there as well. The perimeter of the airport was surrounded by tall trees.

"You remember that incident where one of the flying club members crashed into the trees a few years ago? That was me. I missed runway and landed in the trees." The flying club had been ousted from the airport after the accident for fear of danger to the surrounding residents.

The MFM fellow office was located in the back of Bob's lab space. One day, Andrea, one of the first-year fellows, came to my office to tell me that Bob had come to talk with her about personal issues he was having with his wife. She was not sure what to do about it but wanted to bring it to my attention. I called Bob into my office.

"I hear you may be needing some outside advice for some personal issues. Here is a number to call for mental health services here at the university if you need it. I really think you should take advantage of these services," I said.

He thanked me and took the number. A week later, Bob called me to let me know that he would not be coming in for a few days because he had been in the hospital overnight. Two days later, I was in the ultrasound unit when my secretary called.

"There are two police officers here that want to talk with you."

"Be right there," I replied not having a clue what this was all about. When I arrived to my office, two plain clothes detectives were waiting for me.

"Does Bob work for you?" they asked.

"Sure, he just called me a few days ago to let me know he would need a few days off," I replied.

"We're sorry to tell you this, but Bob has been involved in a mass murder/suicide this morning."

I had to sit down. As the story unfolded, I was told that Bob had been admitted to our university psychiatric hospital for an overnight observation. He was released the following morning. He returned home to get a gun, walked several miles through the woods to his estranged wife's house, and shot her, her boyfriend, and two of his own children. A third child with spina bifida was in a wheelchair at the front of the house waiting for the school bus. When the bus driver heard the shots, he grabbed this boy and put him on the bus. Bob then turned the gun on himself. The detective asked if they could have access to Bob's work computer, which I granted. An email was found where Bob replied in the affirmative for an invitation from me for a barbecue scheduled at my house the following weekend.

The whole event was overwhelming. I learned three weeks later that his family was so angry at Bob that no one had made funeral arrangements. I decided I would have him cremated but a family member finally did come forth to have Bob buried.

I thought the entire incident was behind me when about a month later I received a call from the emergency room.

"There is a woman down here asking if she can come speak to you. She says she is one of Bob's daughters from a previous marriage and she would like to find out what happened," the nurses said.

I decided not to meet with her. I called the detectives instead.

17

What They Don't Teach You in Medical School/Resident Duty Hours/Dwindling State Budgets

My second-born daughter did not meet her developmental milestones when it came to motor function. Termed *congenital hypotonia* by a developmental pediatrician, my wife put her into dance classes at an early age. While all the other little five-year-old girls were waving to their parents at the annual recital, my daughter was concentrating on her *first position* presentation. Perfecting her dance technique as a ballet dancer became a true passion. She regularity attended classes at our local studio and would attend summer program intensives in Florida, Virginia, Texas, and even Italy. Eventually she would attend a high school for the performing arts and later dance as a novice for the Austin ballet.

When she was about eight years old, repetitive *en pointe* positioning of her feet (standing on the tips of the toes) led to extreme pain in her right ankle. My wife took her to an orthopedist that cared for the local professional ballet company. Dr. Jones diagnosed *os trigonum syndrome*—a rare condition in which some individuals have an extra *sesamoid* (accessory) bone located behind their *Achilles tendon*. Most of us do not even know if we have one of these, but when a ballet dancer goes *en pointe*, this rubs on the back of their tendon and causes extreme pain. The orthopedist recommended surgery. Only my wife had met him during the pre-operative visits. At the last visit, Jones told her he would come out and meet us in the pre-operative area before the surgery. This was a considered a standard courtesy between physicians and their patients in most instances. He then told my wife he would go back to the operating room with my daughter.

The morning of surgery, my daughter received her pre-operative meds and then was pulled weeping from her mother's arms as she was taken back on a stretcher into the operating room. I could see the anger in my wife's eyes—no orthopod. We headed off to the waiting room. About ninety minutes later, a tall muscular physician emerged into the room, surgical cap in place with a surgical mask around this neck.

"Is that him?" I asked my wife as I began to stand.

"Sit down," she instructed me. "Let him come over here."

Within a few minutes he managed to identify my wife and find his way over to us.

"Your daughter did fine," he said with a grin.

My wife stood up abruptly. "You told me that you were going to see us in the pre-operative area. You didn't show. They took my daughter back to surgery crying hysterically," she said.

"I didn't know that you wanted to see me before the surgery. The nurses didn't tell me this," he replied.

"The nurses shouldn't have to tell you that. And don't blame the nurses for your lack of compassion," my wife responded.

The surgeon just stood there dumbfounded—no apology, no regret. He simply turned and walked away.

There are many things they teach you in medical school and residency—the course of the median nerve in the arm in anatomy class and how to perform a hysterectomy on the gynecology clinical service. But, what is not often taught is the way to relate to patients. Even worse, we as physicians are not taught to apologize when we are wrong. The whole episode was a valuable life lesson for me.

Several months later, I was on service making rounds with the OB-GYN residents to see the postpartum patients at our hospital. One of my private patients had a *missed abortion* (the fetus had died early in the pregnancy but had not been expelled from her womb). I had scheduled her for a *dilation and curettage (D&C)*. The service was unusually busy that day and I was running behind for the scheduled operating time.

I called down to the pre-operative nurse to explain the situation.

"I will be there shortly. Don't let them take her back until I get to see her," I said.

At this point in my career, it was my routine practice to see my patients in the pre-operative area before they were taken back for surgery. After all, didn't they deserve to know that the doctor they trusted was going to show up for the procedure? After completing rounds, I headed down to Labor and Delivery to find my patient. When I arrived in the pre-operative area, my patient was missing in action.

The nurse informed me that the attending anesthesiologist had insisted we get started on time. "I told him you were running behind but he didn't seem to care," she replied.

I headed over to the operating room where I found my patient already asleep with her legs in stirrups. I was irate!

"Did the nurse not inform you I was running behind?" I asked the anesthesiologist.

"Yeah, but no one else comes to see their patients before surgery so I figured it was OK to take her back and get started. After all we have a busy surgical schedule today," he replied.

"DON'T you ever pull this prank off again with my patients. You have no right. What would you think if this was your wife and I had not seen her before surgery?" I replied.

He looked at me sheepishly over the drapes at the head of the bed. He did not respond. I performed the D&C without problems.

When my patient awoke in the recovery room, I apologized for not getting to see her in the pre-op area. I blamed no one but myself. This would be the last patient that I did not see before one of my surgeries.

One of the biggest changes in residency training was implemented during this time. In 1984, Libby Zion, a freshman student at Bennington College, was admitted to New York Hospital[70]. On an antidepressant medication, she was sedated with a second narcotic medication that resulted in a little-known drug interaction. This caused her to have a high fever that ultimately resulted in a cardiac arrest and her untimely death. Libby's primary physician had admitted her but her in-house care was supervised by an intern and a second-year resident who were caring for forty additional patients that night.

Her father, a prominent attorney in New York, authored an op-ed in the *New York Times* calling into question the supervision and long work hours of the resident physicians at the teaching hospital. The Manhattan District attorney's office sent the case to a grand jury for consideration of murder charges. This in itself was unusual as most cases of medical error that result in the death of a patient are usually tried in civil court as *medical malpractice*. The intern and resident were later charged with thirty-eight counts of gross negligence. The case was sent to the *New York State Board for Professional Medical Conduct* whose final conclusion was that none of the charges were supported by the evidence. In an unusual move, the *New York State Board of Reagents* did not accept the Medical Board's conclusion and sanctioned the two residents for acts of gross negligence. In 1991, an appeals court overturned this ruling and cleared the records of these two physicians. In a latter civil malpractice case, the family of Libby Zion was awarded $375,000 for pain and suffering.

As a result of this very public case, the New York State Health Commissioner called for an ad-hoc committee to make recommendations on resident work hours. Later known as the *Bell Commission*, its final conclusions were published in 1989[71]. Their recommendations included:

- Residents were not allowed to work more than eighty hours/week.

- No more than twenty-four consecutive hours could be worked.

- Supervision by an on-site attending physician must be present at all times.

The rules were adopted by the state of New York in 1989. Fourteen years later in 2003, the *Accreditation Council for Medical Education*

(ACGME) adopted an expanded set of rules for all residency training programs in the U.S.. Additional rules included:

- The eighty-hour weekly limit in duty hours could be averaged over a four-week period.

- A ten-hour rest period was required between duty periods and after call nights.

- A twenty-four-hour limit on continuous duty. An additional six hours was allowed at the hospital for caring for patients admitted in the previous twenty-four hours or to participate in educational activities.

- No new patients could be cared for by the resident after the twenty-four-hour period.

- One day in seven had to be free of clinical or educational activities averaged over a four- week period.

- In-house call could not be more frequent than one in three nights averaged over four weeks.

The *ACGME* rules have been modified twice since their original inception. In 2011, the rules were revised to limit duty hours for interns to sixteen continuous hours[72]. In 2017, this rule was changed back to allow twenty-four hours of continuous work by interns. In addition, interns had to be directly supervised by the attending physician[73].

The European Union approved the European Working Directive for resident duty hours in 1998[74]. These included:

- A maximum work week of forty-eight hours (as compared to the eighty-hour U.S. work week).

- An eleven-hour rest period was required between duty periods and after call nights.

- One day in seven or two days in a fourteen-day period had to be free of clinical or educational activities.

- Twenty-minute rest period every six hours.

- Four weeks paid leave annually.

Like many other OB-GYN residency programs, implementation of these new guidelines at our program was problematic. Although attending faculty slept in-house every night, they were reluctant to awaken to supervise the residents with anything but the most difficult of cases. The knowledge that they themselves were not subject to restrictions on *duty hours* reinforced this attitude. In most cases, faculty were assigned to clinical duties the following day. This was necessary to generate sufficient clinical revenue to maintain salaries. As time progressed, Dr. Papel and I reformulated the work schedule of the faculty so that *post-call* attending was allowed to leave by noon the following day.

But the problem still remained as to how to adhere to the *AAMC* resident rules. Deviation from these could lead to probation for the residency program—a black mark for future recruitment of residents. Like many other institutions, a *night float* system was instituted. A team of residents (usually one per each training level) was assigned to work Sunday night through Thursday night from 5 p.m.to 7 a.m. Other residents would cover the day shift and take twenty-four-hour calls on weekends. There were two immediate detrimental effects of this change.

Our residency prided itself on its commitment to education. With the exception of emergency surgery and obstetrical deliveries, outpatient services had been closed after noon on Wednesdays. During that afternoon, grand rounds, morbidity and mortality conference, faculty meetings, and resident and student lectures were scheduled. With the adoption of the night float system, the residents assigned to this rotation would not be able to participate in any of these activities. The second issue that became evident was related to patient care. In the older system, there was one patient turnover each day. One team would care for a patient for the first twenty-four hours and then "pass the baton" to the next team the following morning. With night float, a three *baton passes* occurred. This meant that unless there was significant attention to detail, important clinical items could be missed during *check out rounds*.

As an example, on one occasion, I was called back to assist in a hysterectomy in a patient who had just been delivered of her first baby by C-section. The uterus had developed *atony*, a condition where the muscles in the uterus do not work effectively to contract the uterus down after the baby has been removed. In this scenario, the uterus is "floppy" and the site of the placenta attachment continues to bleed profusely. Various medications like *methergine, prostaglandin,* and *oxytocin* had all been given to help the uterine muscle contract. None seemed to have any effect. To stop the bleeding, we would have to remove the uterus, rendering the patient infertile after having delivered her first child. I felt the situation was so unusual that after the case, I immediately went to review the chart. In the brief presentation to me by the resident staff when I was summoned to the operating room, I had been informed that the patient was admitted twelve hours earlier and had been on an oxytocin infusion to stimulate labor during that time. The cervix had not continued to dilate, so the chief resident had made a diagnosis of *cephalopelvic disproportion* (the baby's head was too big to fit through the patient's pelvis) and a decision was made to deliver the baby by C-section. This all seemed reasonable to me. Then I looked over the nurses' notes. What I discovered was that the patient had not been on *oxytocin* for twelve hours but instead she had been on the medication for thirty-six hours. This was beginning to make sense. The uterus is a muscle and when you administer a drug that makes it contract every three or four minutes for thirty-six hours, it gets tired. Lactic acid builds up in the muscle cells. When you ask it to contract down immediately after the baby has been born, it's is too exhausted to function. The proper management would have been to "rest" the patient after the first day of the *oxytocin* infusion. It was clear that the residents had missed the time course of the *oxytocin* during check-out rounds. The baton had been dropped in this marathon race. As a consequence, the patient had lost her uterus.

Studies on sleep deprivation have indicated that after twenty-four hours, a person has a reaction time equivalent to someone with a blood alcohol level of 0.10%, higher than the legal limit for a *driving under the influence* conviction in most states[75]. One of our OB-GYN residents had received notification from her auto insurance company that they would not renew her policy if she had any additional accidents. On three different occasions when she was driving home after a call night, she stopped at a traffic light. Falling asleep, she would take her foot off the brake and roll into traffic where she was promptly "T-boned" by oncoming cars. Fortunately, she was never seriously injured in these accidents. Her fellow residents teamed up after the third incident and always drove her home *post-call.*

Sleep deprivation studies in medical care are conflicting. A randomized study of surgical interns published in 2016 studied programs that strictly adhered to the *AAMC* rules versus allowing the residency directors to adopt a flexible work schedule[76]. Both arms of the study included a restriction of eighty hours of total duty per week. Flexible schedules with including working *post-call* were not associated with more surgical deaths or complications. Surgical *interns* with flexible schedules reported less dissatisfaction with the continuity of patient care. A more recent study was conducted in a similar fashion and involved internal medicine *interns*[77]. Flexible schedules were not associated with increased patient death or readmissions to the hospital. More importantly, test results of mental alertness while on duty were similar in the flexible work schedule group as compared to the strict *AAMC* guidelines group.

Although residency duty hour restrictions have enabled a better *work–life balan*ce for the current class of residents, the detrimental impact on residency training is evident. Before the new rule, the typical resident worked one hundred hours per week (60% of the one hundred sixty-eight total hours in a week). The restriction to eighty hours meant a loss of 20% of the clinical experience over each year of a four-year OB-GYN residency—the equivalent of almost a calendar year of lost experience. As I pointed out in an earlier chapter, there is no replacement for patient exposure so that the physician in training can begin to recognize patterns of disease presentation and their proper treatment. Adding to this diminished OB-GYN training opportunity is the loss of an extensive pregnant patient population at inner-city hospitals. The annual number of deliveries at the original inner-city hospital where I trained as a fellow was 18,000. Today the two new hospitals in our city (now staffed by two different medical schools) only did a total of 4,200 deliveries in 2021. A fall in the national birth rate is not the explanation for this shift. Most states have improved access to prenatal care by decreasing the income threshold for Medicaid eligibility during pregnancy. This is good for patients. But, it also provides the opportunity to seek the care of private physicians instead of delivering at a teaching hospital.

Leaders in our field are struggling with how to address this problem. *Competencies* have been developed by the *ACGME* requiring residents to keep case logs of patients, and attendings must sign off on their residents' surgical skills. Most programs have developed *simulation labs*—rubber mannequins are used to practice the management of acute situations such as *shoulder dystocia* (the baby's head delivers at the time of a vaginal delivery but the shoulders are impacted, preventing further successful delivery) or *postpartum hemorrhage* (the loss of too much blood after delivery). These efforts can only partially address the loss of clinical experience. Perhaps virtual reality technology much like the vivid scenes produced by the gaming industry will be the future training modality for residents. Other leaders have proposed increasing the length of the OB-GYN residency. This is unlikely to occur for two reasons—the average school debt of residents will have them steer away from programs that require yet another year of low wages. More importantly, hospital budgets cannot afford to add the salaries and benefits of an additional class of residents to their existing programs. Clearly, some modifications to our current methods of residency training will be needed if we are to maintain the level of competency we expect from our healthcare system. Our patients deserve this!

When I arrived to my new department, state funds were paying almost one-third of the budget of the medical school. There was little incentive for the faculty to do more than supervise the residents and bill the state for the care of the indigent patients. Having come from other institutions, Dr. Papel and I knew that a large state subsidy could not be expected to last forever.

About two years after our arrival, the state budget was in trouble due to decreasing tax revenues. This would mean less money for the medical school. The state legislature threatened to take the *indirect expenses* from the National Institutes of Health grants that investigators at the medical school had been awarded. They rationalized that since state tax revenue had partially funded the medical school, the state was entitled to these funds to help balance the budget that year. The *National Institutes of Health (NIH)* is the best funded research institution of any industrialized country, with an annual budget of \$45 billion in 2022[78]. Tax revenue to the federal government is invested in medical research in an effort to improve the health of U.S. citizens. The *NIH* consists of twenty-seven institutes and centers including a research hospital located in Bethesda, Maryland. More than 80% of its budget is used to fund more than 35,000 grants of investigators at medical schools and other universities. Each medical school negotiates the percentage of the basic grant award needed for administrative costs and the costs to maintain facilities, the so-called *indirect expenses*. These monies are used to maintain infrastructure, process grant applications, and hire new research faculty. The percentage of indirect costs vary based on local costs at universities. Some southern schools negotiate an indirect rate of 60%, while some East Coast schools are paid more than 100% in *indirect costs*. Our dean ultimately won the budget battle with the state legislature that year—he threatened to close down the research endeavors at the medical school if the *indirects* were removed from his budget.

Research grants awarded by the NIH are used as one parameter in the ranking of U.S. medical schools in the annual *U.S. News and World Report*[79]. This means that medical schools are committed to research endeavors. This requires additional commitment of monies to allow these investigators to have *protected time* to undertake the research. The cap on physician clinical salaries by the *NIH* in 2022 was \$203,700. This is less than the typical base salary offered to even the most junior of faculty necessary to compete with private practice opportunities. Therefore, if a physician investigator is involved in a 20% effort (one day each week for research), the medical school must make up the percentage of their base salary and benefits not covered by the *NIH* grant. Medical schools provide cost sharing during other

NIH research projects as well. Dr. Papel felt that we should attempt to become a member of the *NIH-funded Maternal-Fetal Research Network.* Membership in this network is considered a prestigious distinction of an MFM Division. The current network consists of twelve academic institutions distributed throughout the country. Clinical trials are planned by the members and conducted on a large scale to improve the care of pregnant women. Joining this network is no small task. The application has to include a complete description of the institution's research infrastructure as well as an original research proposal that may later be used by the network.

Despite Dr. Papel's objection, I named Dr. Thomas as the *principal investigator* for the application, with me serving in the capacity of *co-investigator*. After all he had demonstrated the most commitment to obstetrical research in the MFM Division. A senior research nurse that I had recruited from my previous medical school was assigned to be the lead research nurse. The grant would pay for 20% of Dr. Thomas's salary, one research nurse, and a data entry person. All other funds would be based on each study patient enrolled in the ongoing clinical trials for the network. We were fortunate to be awarded an invitation to join the *NIH MFM network*—a real feather in the cap for the department and the Division.

A short time later, I met with Karen, our lead research nurse. "I need to hire two more research nurses. I cannot get all this NIH paperwork done and find patients for the studies at the same time," she told me.

"How long do you think the Division will need to come up with the funds for their salaries?" I asked.

"About a year," she answered. I had enough experience in academic medicine at this point in my career to know that it's better to multiply such projections by two-to-threefold. I was right—we broke even on the network grant two years later—our Division's monetary commitment to improve the health of pregnant women in America!

A new women's hospital was being constructed on our campus. It was time to, as Dr. Papel used to say, "Put some other eggs in the basket" to diversify the income sources for the department. So, we set out to develop more of a private patient presence with the new hospital coming on board. All faculty would be asked to see private obstetrical patients two half days a week. Deliveries would be covered by the attending who was on call or the attending assigned to the service each week. A "country-partner" scheme was proposed—attendings would team up in pairs and cover each other's clinic days when their partner was assigned to the OB inpatient service.

At first there was general acceptance by the Division. However, there was one notable exception. Dr. Thomas had graduated from the residency at our institution. He had approached the Chairman at the time to stay on as an *Assistant Professor* but was told that they did not have a general OB-GYN Division so he would have to do fellowship training in a specialty. He chose an MFM fellowship. Thomas never really functioned as an MFM. He had no skills in ultrasound and continued to practice routine gynecology, something most MFM's stop doing. But his biggest issue was that he felt there was no reason to change the way things had been done at the university since he was a resident in OB-GYN. Dr. Thomas traveled quite a bit, which is not uncommon among academic physicians. The problem again comes down to balancing budgets.

When an academic physician gives grand rounds at another institution, their salary continues to be paid by the medical school where they hold an appointment. The other institution defrays the costs of travel and pays a small honorarium to the physician. Long-standing tradition dictates that the physician gets to keep this honorarium for the effort required to prepare and give the presentation. These presentations are considered a routine part of academic medicine. They serve to educate the medical community while enhancing the reputation of the parent institution and the physician themselves. The problem is that when an attending physician travels excessively, the Division begins to subsidize these efforts. Since the more senior attendings receive the most invitations (and since they are earning the higher salaries), this places a significant burden on entry-level attendings. Dr. Papel and I met and decided the best way to deal with this was to ask all the attendings to cover an equal number of private clinics. If they traveled, they would be required to schedule "make-up" clinics on days when they were not assigned to other clinical services.

Dr. Thomas did not like this concept. Every quarter, the attendings would be given a projected number of clinics they should attempt to schedule. Vacation time and allotted time for outside academic endeavors were taken into account. This was deemed the new compensation plan which included a 10% hold-back for bad behavior as determined by the Chairman. Thomas continued to travel unabated so I decided to audit his clinics. Much to my dismay, he fell almost ten clinics short in one quarter. Our clinic software deleted the previous quarter's clinic schedule on a rolling basis, so I had to ask for the tape back-up to look at these.

I called for a meeting with Dr. Thomas.

"I looked back at last quarter and you fell short by ten clinics. How do you explain that?" I asked. I fully expected Thomas would admit to this shortcoming and agree to rectify it the next quarter.

Instead he confronted me. "How do you know that I didn't do those clinics?" he asked.

Well I looked at the computer records for the dates you reported to me that you saw patients and there were none scheduled that day," I said.

"Well the computer is wrong," he replied.

"That's not possible for every one of these ten clinics," I said. When the patient checks in, they are logged into the system. There were no patients seen on those days."

"Well, those appointments are not even displayed in our computer system anymore," he interjected.

"Yes, but the hospital keeps electronic records for years of these appointments," I answered (it was clear that Thomas was not aware of how computerized systems worked at the institution). "Again, are you insisting that you saw patients on those days?" I asked.

"Yep," he responded.

I consulted Dr. Papel and we decided the best course of action was to implement the 10% hold-back on salary for the involved quarter for Dr. Thomas. He was of course furious. He decided to complain to the Dean of the medical school. The Dean was a reasonable man and decided to convene a review panel of senior attendings from outside the department. Dr. Papel and I had to appear before the committee. I provided the panel a copy of the Dr. Thomas' alleged clinics and a copy of the electronic records of the clinic schedules for those days. The panel reported to the Dean that the actions of the Chair of OB-GYN were upheld.

Thomas was even more furious and confronted the Dean. "I've been at this institution for a long time. Longer than you have. I know people. I'm taking this to the President of the university."

The Dean responded, "Please proceed. He will only support my decision after he learns about the investigation. You are wasting your time."

Thomas finally accepted the chair's decision for the hold-back. He scheduled all the clinics asked of him thereafter.

Architects who design hospitals never work or sleep in them. They should. The new Women's Hospital was rising from the foundation when I had the opportunity to look over the plans. The new director of obstetrical ultrasound I had recruited was particularly interested in the ultrasound suites. Before her arrival, I had implemented several upgrades to the current ultrasound unit. We had rented new state-of-the-art machines connected them to a computer network to store images and create reports that could be faxed to referring physicians the same day they were completed. Previously, ultrasounds were stored on VHS videotapes and reports were dictated, sent to transcription, and mailed out to physicians more than two weeks later. We were a product of our own success. The number of ultrasound referrals increased by almost 30%.

Dr. Wopler and I decided to make life-size paper cutouts of the footprints of all the equipment in each ultrasound room. We then grabbed flashlights and one night like Watergate burglars we navigated our way through the steel framing at the construction site of the new hospital to the future ultrasound suites. After laying the cutouts on the floor, we immediately recognized a problem. All of our sonographers were trained to scan right-handed. This meant the ultrasound machine would have to be located on the patient's right side and the computer would need to be next to it. But when we laid out the room, the wash sink was on the wall behind the ultrasound machine where all the power outlets would have to be located. In order to propose a correction to the construction, we divulged our burglar-like affair.

We were banished from the building but the power and plumbing were modified and moved down the wall in all the ultrasound suites.

Other issues were identified and addressed. We had a chance to re-design the headwalls in the labor rooms to better accommodate a future EMR workstation.

I then discovered that the bathroom doors in the labor rooms appeared to have been mounted backwards—the door opened towards the front of the room blocking the nurse's view of a patient that might have fallen or fainted in the bathroom doorway. The door should have opened against the wall allowing easy access by the nurse in the event of an emergency. I was told this was too expensive to change at the advanced state of construction.

And then there was the issue of the emergency elevator in the back of the new hospital that allowed pregnant women seen in the emergency room to be brought straight up to Labor and Delivery. I thought this was an excellent feature. There was only one small wrinkle—why wasn't the elevator shaft extended one more floor upward? This was the location of the undelivered pregnant women who were hospitalized with medical problems or bleeding. Would it happen that a patient might need to be acutely transferred down to Labor and Delivery in an emergency? Again, I was told this would be too expensive to change at this late stage in the construction process.

A few months after the hospital had opened, my fears were confirmed. A patient on the *antepartum* (undelivered OB patients) floor with a *placenta previa* began bleeding profusely. She would need to be moved to Labor and Delivery for an emergency C-section. We would need to use the passenger elevators at the front of the hospital to transfer the patient. We had previously thought about the need for an emergency key to control access and had secured one and attached it to a souvenir football helmet so it was easy to find. The nurses grabbed the key and wheeled the patient in her bed to the passenger elevator. But we had never drilled this before. The bed was too long for the elevator. Someone managed to find a transport stretcher and we moved the patient over to it. Then we headed down the elevator.

Other issues manifested themselves after we opened the new building. The second night after we opened, I was on call in-house. The chief resident called me at around midnight. "I need to switch call rooms with you. I can't sleep in this resident call room," she said.

"Why?" I asked.

"Come over for a minute," was the answer. I went to her call room and sat on the bed. "Wait," she said.

A few minutes later there was distant swooshing sound followed shortly afterwards by a loud rushing noise. The architect had designed the pneumatic tube system used to transport blood samples from the upper floors of the hospital to the lab to be located in the wall of the chief resident's call room!

More administrative tasks would lie ahead. Soon after my arrival, Dr. Papel asked me to address programmatic issues with the MFM fellowship program. Dr. Thomas was the Director, at least that's what the last application stated. He had done little to bring the training program in line with new guidelines from *ABOG*. Fellows were basically assigned to provide most of the clinical care on Labor and Delivery and the antepartum unit. Off-service rotations to increase their clinical expertise were not part of the program and research efforts were bare bones. I was actually surprised that the fellowship had not been reviewed and placed on probation. Since the president of *ABOG* was the long-standing Director of the department's MFM Division, I figured this had allowed *ABOG* to "look the other way" when it came to the organization of our training program. At Dr. Papel's insistence, I named myself the fellowship Director and

proceeded to submit a new application. The structure was re-orga-
nized and new pathways developed that would allow a fellow to
obtain a concurrent *Masters in Public Health* or a *Masters in Health Care
Administration* at the neighboring state school of public health. We
passed our subsequent site visit with flying colors.

Dr. Papel was truly a woman of vision. Before my arrival, she
had negotiated a salary line from the Dean of the medical school to
recruit a Director for a new center. Its main goal was to improve the
health of pregnant women and their unborn children in the state. We
were fortunate to recruit Lucille, a social worker with a PhD from
her position in the Northeast. She had a track record for being able
to raise funding. Dr. Papel named me as the obstetrical co-Director
for the center; I recruited a pediatric cardiologist to be the pediatric
co-Director. Together the three of us would provide the leadership for
the new center. Lucille orchestrated a strategic planning process that
involved ten different committees of interested parties at the medical
school. The main goal was to get buy-in for the new center. Ultimately
the planning process developed a name—*the Center for Maternal and
Infant Health*. Lucille applied for two grants from local non-for-profit
foundations and secured over three million dollars in funding. We
were able to hire a full-time IT consultant to build a website and a
unique database. Several nurse coordinators were hired to provide
care coordination for pregnant women with complications sent from
rural hospitals from around the state. Pregnant patients with unborn
children with birth defects were guided through the difficult process
of meeting with various pediatric consultants to learn what would
happen to their babies once they delivered. At the end of the grant
funding periods, Lucille left the center and we were lucky enough
to recruit the Director of the local chapter of the March of Dimes to
be the executive Director of our Center—Sally. Almost twelve years
later, the center continues to address such key issues in pregnancy as

progesterone availability for women at risk for premature delivery, smoking cessation, and postpartum depression.

Obstetrics can be a constant challenge to keep up with the public demand for a holistic birthing experience. Until the later 1800s, obstetrical deliveries occurred in the home with the assistance of a family member or a midwife. The turn of the 19th century in the U.S. saw a move to hospital-based deliveries with a new caregiver—the physician obstetrician as the attendant.

Many changes in OB practice have occurred in recent years including a return to the home deliveries. A recent study of home births in Oregon noted a 2.4-fold increase in the incidence of newborn death during birth through the first month of life[80]. Home births were more often associated with newborn seizures and the need for oxygen support by a ventilator for these infants as well. Because of the risks, the *American College of Obstetricians and Gynecologists (ACOG)* has taken a position against home delivers. Other recent practices include *placentophagy*—saving the afterbirth after a delivery to have it freeze dried and placed in medication capsules. Touted by the Hollywood community as a cure for postpartum depression, *ACOG* does not advocate this practice. More recently, the issue of *vaginal seeding* has come into vogue. In this situation, vaginal secretions are swabbed from the vagina and then applied the newborn's face at the time of elective C-section. This is proposed to allow the normal exposure to maternal bacteria to enhance the development of newborn immunity. The current statement from *ACOG* does not support this practice due to the risk for infections in the newborn. In my time as Chief of Obstetrics, underwater birth was also making its debut into obstetrical practice.

I received a call one day to ask me to come to Labor and Delivery. "A patient has just arrived and is filling up her birthing tub and we are not sure what to do," said the nurse.

When I arrived a few minutes later, I entered the labor room to find a metal frame assembled a few feet inside the doorway of the labor room. The frame was about five by five feet square. Attached to the frame was a plastic liner so that the whole apparatus appeared to resemble one of those above-ground swimming pools for the backyard. A plastic hose had been connected to the sink in the room and was filling the tub with water. It was already about half-full. I talked with the OB patient who was presenting with early contractions.

"Did we know you were coming with the portable tub?" I inquired.

"I did inform my midwife that I was planning to use it. She said it would be OK," she responded.

"Well we really haven't been faced with this before. I have some concerns with the tub. For example, how will we empty it?" I asked.

"That's easy," she said. "I have a hose with a pump that comes with it that will empty it into the toilet."

I offered several other concerns. "How will we monitor the heart rate of the baby during labor?" I asked.

She of course had done her homework and had an answer for this as well. "I have a waterproof hand-held Doppler device that the midwife was planning to use," she responded.

I was running out of reasons why she should not use this tub.

"Well I am concerned about the floor support for this extra weight (turns out that water weighs eight pounds/gallon and the tub with an estimated capacity of 500 gallons would have a total weight equal to two tons). And then there was the issue of a potential break in the liner that would result in a massive biohazard spill of blood and other bodily fluids. I really don't think we are going to be able to let you use this tub", I finally said.

The patient and her husband were upset with my proclamation.

"We do have a Jacuzzi tub in the room where you can labor," I offered. This did not seem to appease the couple.

I heard later they talked their midwife into letting them deliver in the Jacuzzi tub. Later our Labor and Delivery working group met and discussed the issues. The architect agreed that the structure of the floors was suspect to accommodate the weight of the water in these tubs. We decided we would not allow patients to use them. A few months later, the editor of the journal *Pediatrics* wrote an editorial in response to two cases of drowning in newborn infants at the time of delivery. He felt the practice of underwater births should be abandoned.

It was time for Dr. Papel's five-year review as Chair of the Department. All Division Directors were asked to prepare reports of the accomplishments of their divisions and would testify in front of the reviewers. This seemed relatively easy for me—we had made great strides in establishing private patient services while enhancing our research efforts. I was one of the last Division Directors to appear before the committee. Within a few minutes, it was soon apparent that I would be the target of their questions. I could only assume that I was the subject of the discussion with the other Division Directors during their appearances. After all, I was the only Division Director Dr. Papel had recruited. And she had charged me with bringing major changes to the obstetrical service.

The faculty in most of the other divisions had remained unchanged during this time period. This had not been the case in the MFM Division. The two former senior faculty had decided to change to part-time positions, sharing one salary line. Neither wanted to take call or staff Labor and Delivery any longer. This left only the outpatient clinics in need of staffing. This was easy for Dr. Botts— he enjoyed seeing patients. However, this was not the case for Dr. Seth. His initial career was based in the armed services and he had "retired" to run the MFM Division for nineteen years. He would later become the chair of the *American Board of Obstetrics and Gynecology* and even be called upon to chair the first maternal research network sponsored by the *National Institutes of Health*. Seeing all the changes occurring in the Division he had once created in his own image was difficult. Dr. Seth did not relish seeing patients in clinic. Later with the retirement of Dr. Botts, he was appointed to an assistant dean-ship at the medical school in order to maintain his full-time position at the medical school.

Other changes in the original MFM faculty would also take place. Two would move to a nearby medical school—a common practice in academic medicine. New faculty would be recruited. Dr. James, a long-time colleague and friend, would join our faculty to establish a fetal center and to upgrade the genetic testing laboratory that the department ran for obstetrical patients from around the state. Dr. Wopler would become the matriarch of the ultrasound unit— hiring a team of excellent sonographers that she would protect at all costs. Dr. Bonny would be recruited from a nearby medical school to begin infectious disease research in conjunction with the neighbor-ing state dental school. There a dentist was attempting to understand the role of poor dentition and its relationship to premature delivery. Dr. Comier would later be appointed Chair of OB-GYN at another little ivy medical school where I had previously done my OB-GYN residency training.

Looking back, I am sure that the rapidity of the changes in the MFM Division was poorly received at an institution that had seen little change in over twenty years. At times I was probably blind to the political capital that was lost in accomplishing the goals asked of me by my chair.

At the five-year review, I was asked, "Do you have any regrets on the way you were doing things in your Division?"

Once when I was struggling with a difficult issue as a Division Director, I consulted a long-standing Division Director at a New York medical school.

"Ken he said, if you are making fair decisions, you should not have any problems sleeping each night. If your head hits the pillow and you do not spend time re-thinking all the decisions you made that day, you're probably doing the job you should be doing for the Division."

I knew that I normally fell asleep within five minutes those days. I told that story to the committee to answer their question.

One year later, Dr. Papel elected to leave our department to become the Dean at another medical school. She advised the Dean at our current medical school that I would be the best candidate as the acting Chair since I knew the most about the departmental operations. I was summoned to the Dean's office.

"Dr. Papel tells me that you are the man for the job as the acting chair of the OB-GYN department."

"I appreciate the offer," I responded. "But I don't think this would be good for the department. I am not sure that I would be well accepted by the current faculty."

"Well, do you think the retired chair of the surgery department could do the job?"

"I don't think this is would be great for residency recruitment."

"Who would you suggest then?" he asked.

"Well, Dr. Seth is well respected by the current faculty. In addition, he has been the acting Chair in the past for the department."

The Dean named Dr. Seth as the acting Chair. A month later, Dr. Seth called me into his office for a discussion.

"Ken, I would like to offer you a research sabbatical."

"I appreciate the offer at this point in my career, but we still have some major projects in the Division that need my attention," I replied.

He then handed me a book about the history of the missionary efforts of the Jesuits that he asked me to read. On further introspection, I missed these cues. Clearly, Dr. Lo felt it his responsibility to replace me before a new chair was selected. Several candidates interviewed for the chair position and the Dean selected a candidate who was the Director of oncology at a neighboring medical school.

A few days later, I was called to the assistant dean's office. I really was at a loss as to what the agenda might be. When I arrived, Dr. Lo was sitting on the couch but would not make eye contact with me.

The assistant dean spoke "Ken we would like you to resign as the Director of the MFM Division."

I was shocked.

"As a tenured professor, you can remain as a member of the Division." I remained perplexed.

"So, you want me to save face by resigning?" I said.

"We think it would be better this way," he responded.

"Not sure that I want to resign. I think I would rather have you say that you just asked me to step down. Let's call it what it is and not sugarcoat it." And oh, by the way, do you want me to step down as the fellowship Director too?" I asked.

The dean looked at me perplexed at having not been briefed by Dr. Lo on the many roles that I played in the department.

"Yes," he responded.

"And the co-Director of the Center for Maternal and Child Health? And the clinical Director of the obstetrical service at the Women's Hospital?" I inquired.

"Yes, to all those roles," the dean answered.

"Just checking," I replied. Having received one of the most significant setbacks in my academic career, I stood up and left the Dean's office. An email was sent out by the Dean within five minutes of my departure, announcing that I had been asked to step down.

The next day I received an email from the Dean re-instating me in the role of co-Director of the Center for Maternal and Infant Health.

The new chair arrived and I asked for a meeting with him.

"We barely met during your interview process. I really wish we would have had the opportunity to discuss my role in your vision of the department. I would have respected you more if you would not have counted on the hearsay of the other faculty to have the acting chair ask me to step down before your arrival."

Later, several candidates for MFM Division Director were interviewed and the Chair decided to hire a former MFM fellow who was now an Associate Professor at a neighboring medical school—a return to the old guard.

When I asked her during her interview why she wanted this job, she replied, "I always wanted to come back to this state. That way my children can go to these great universities with in-state tuition."

I thought the answer showed a lack of vision.

I had given eight years of my life to the program. Dr. Papel and I had struggled to bring the Division around and we had succeeded on several fronts. The next insult came when my former secretary, now the administrative assistant for the chair, called my office.

"We need you to move to a smaller office in the back of the MFM suite so that the new Director can have your office," she said.

"Why is that?" I asked.

"The office across from me is the same size and there is an *Assistant Professor* there. I am a *tenured full Professor*."

"The new Director wants to move into your office because she always remembers Dr. Seth being there as the Division Director."

"Oh, I see, and she could not talk to me about this? I'll get to packing up my books."

The final insult came after a British film crew had come to our institution to do a documentary on a new fetal surgical procedure we were doing. During the course of the week we spent with them, we even took them to the top of the hospital to shoot views of the university. The segment appeared in prime-time television on the 20-20 show. We never received any acknowledgment from the new Division Director or Chair. It was time to leave! Several of the faculty approached me about an exit party. Given the recent circumstances, I thought it better to decline. I did receive a commemorative captain's chair with a plaque on the back indicating my years of service.

One of my favorite mini-series is *Lonesome Dove*. A former Texas ranger decides to take his rag-tag group of cowboys on a cattle drive starting in Texas to establish the first cattle ranch in Montana. Along the way, many of his colleagues lose their lives for various reasons. In the final scene, McCall has returned to Texas to fulfill a promise to one of his dearest friends "to bury him in a little pecan orchard near a creek where he used to picnic with a woman he loved." When he returns to the Texas town where the whole journey began, he is confronted by a reporter.

"They say you are a man of vision," the reporter says to him.

McCall looks over the horizon, ponders for a moment, and then replies, "A man of vision you say. Hella of a vision."

I had no regrets after I left my position as the MFM Division Director. I had accomplished my vision and succeeded in what my dad had taught me, "Always leave it a little better place than when you arrived."

18

Moving On/A New Chair/ A New Woman's Hospital

I had recruited Dr. James to our MFM Division to develop a fetal surgery program. He and I had been friends for many years and we had shared a passion for fetal medicine—an evolving field. A study of an exciting new laser procedure for the treatment of a complication of unborn identical twins was presented at an international meeting we both attended in Switzerland[81]. Identical twins share a common placenta and there are connecting blood vessels between the two in almost all cases. In about 10%–15% of cases, blood begins to move from one twin to the other. The *donor* twin gets stuck in its sac against the wall of the uterus as it stops producing urine. This is called *oligo-hydramnios* (decreased amniotic fluid). The *recipient* twin experiences excessive urine production in an effort to prevent the development of congestive heart failure. A massive amount of amniotic fluid builds up in its sac (*polyhydramnios*). Without treatment, over 90% of these pregnancies are lost. After recruiting Dr. James to join our Division, I made arrangements for him to go to Europe to observe the procedure in Paris and Leuven. In this procedure, a small telescope (*fetoscope*) is placed into the amniotic sac of the recipient twin and the problematic vessels on the placenta are located and spot welded with a laser. But now it was apparent that the support from our new Chair (an oncologist) had dissipated and it was time to see where we could continue our efforts in this new field. James went North to Chicago to propose a *fetal center* at a major medical institution there. I returned to my alma mater in the Southwest. Chicago rejected the proposal but the Chair of Pediatrics at my former institution was interested. There were ongoing plans for his large pediatric hospital to move into the obstetrical business. Most pediatric hospitals are free-standing and are only affiliated with a nearby adult hospital that provides obstetrical services. This would be unique for a pediatric hospital to offer an OB delivery service. A *fetal center* would fit well with this plan. Several issues surfaced as we began our negotiations.

Dr. Lo, who was the Chairman of OB-GYN when I left the medical school eight years earlier to move to the East Coast, remained as the Chair of the current department. We were told however that we would not be meeting with him because he would soon be replaced by a new acting Chair, Dr. Green.

Since my departure, MFM faculty had continued to leave the department so that there were no longer any faculty remaining in the MFM Division. In order to be recruited, we would have to commit not only to establish a *fetal center* but we would be required to assist with the care of pregnant patients with medical complications. Although I felt comfortable with this, James did not. Although board-certified as a Maternal–Fetal specialist as a *Doctor of Osteopathy (D.O.)*, most of his training and clinical experience had been related to prenatal ultrasound and genetics. In the end, I agreed to provide maternal consultations at the inner-city hospital where I had once supervised the OB service, until more MFM faculty could be recruited. James would be protected to work primarily at the *fetal center*.

Prior to our arrival, two young pediatric surgeons had declared themselves to be the co-Directors of a newly established *fetal center* at the pediatric hospital. Due to the lack of affiliated MFM faculty, the *center* had been experiencing difficulty in gaining traction. During our initial meetings, we informed them that we were not interested in titles but would rather collaborate for the success of the center. It came time for *the napkin*—deciding the conditions for our recruitment. Dr. Green had been recruited as the acting Chair of OB-GYN from his clinical appointment in private practice. Well respected by the private physicians in the medical center, he was perceived as the consummate Southern gentleman. But Dr. Green had never worked in academic medicine. His inclination was to make recruitment promises to James and I "on a handshake." I knew better. He might not be the Chairman in a few short months. We were uprooting our families to move to a new city and we wanted a five-year contract. Having done this in the past in my role as an MFM division Director, I decided to write the recruitment letters for both James and me. After several versions went back and forth using track changes in a Word document, we finally came to an agreement on the conditions of our employment.

The political environment between the private hospitals and the medical school was quite tumultuous at the time. The administration of the large adult hospital in the medical center that had been affiliated with the medical school for almost fifty years decided to sever its financial ties with the school. The new Dean of the medical school wanted to build an outpatient surgery center (thereby diverting cases from the hospital) in an effort to improve clinical revenues. This did not sit well with the hospital. The subsequent "divorce" would cost the medical school more than twenty million dollars in annual support. The name of the medical school was removed from all of the facades of the office buildings. Without this support, most of the departments of the medical school were now in financial trouble and many full-time faculty would leave the school for private practice. This was not the case with the Department of Pediatrics. The long-standing Chairman had an excellent rapport with his residents; his department even paid for their parking. Many would stay in the city after their training to develop primary care pediatric practices. He had organized them into a network to refer all their patients that needed subspecialty care to the ever-growing pediatric hospital. The pediatric hospital first opened in early 1950s. Due to limited funding, a decision was made to build one structure—a pediatric hospital and an adjoining adult hospital. Laundry services and even the dining room for patients would be shared. There would be one board of Directors for both hospitals. Years later, separate boards of directors were created. As we arrived at our new institution, another political upheaval was occurring.

The adjoining adult hospital in the medical center that had provided obstetrical services since its very establishment decided to close its obstetrical service. Of note, Karen and I had delivered all three of our daughters in the same labor room at this hospital. The OB service was no longer making money for the hospital—all revenue being generated by the admission of premature babies was going to the children's hospital next door. And that hospital did not want to profit share.

Needing a place for the pregnant patients to deliver, the children's hospital elected to buy the obstetrical service as an interim solution. All of the obstetrical nurses were transferred to their staff and the hospital would rent the Labor and Delivery space and the postpartum ward at the adult hospital. This arrangement would not last long. Given its lucrative financial status, the pediatric hospital decided to purchase adjacent land.

The CEO of the children's hospital told me, "It costs me what Park Place would cost in a Monopoly game."

The plan would be for the children's hospital to build their own obstetrical hospital to support their pediatric service—the first venture of this magnitude in the U.S. The children's hospital was always great at public relations. The implosion of the hotel on the newly acquired property occurred with great fanfare. We were all invited to the event. A young oncology patient was even allowed to push a fake plunger to start the explosions to implode the building. The competing for-profit women's hospital in town was rumored to support a story of a homeless person having been seen in the building just before the demolition. This was highly unlikely since all of the metal stairwells in the hotel had been removed for recycling. In addition, the area had been cordoned off for several days before the implosion and police had inspected the site. In any event, the local news stations broadcasted the searches by the cadaver dogs—no body was found.

James and I would work overtime to establish the new *fetal center*. We traveled around a four-state area and met all of the MFMs that might refer a patient for fetal surgery. Based on my previous experiences with the new hospital at my last position, I offered to assist in the planning of the structure of the new women's hospital. Being busy with clinical activities most days, the planning meetings were scheduled after hours. The planning committee started by deciding whether the building should be squared off with the adjoining streets or whether it should be angled for better visualization from the surrounding buildings. We decided on angling the building. Next came the decision where to place the elevator shafts.

"Why are we talking about this?" I inquired.

"They are the most dense structures of the building. Where we put them dictates how the inside of the building is laid out," responded the architect.

Karen and I spent long hours in planning meetings. We even went to a local warehouse where the architects had constructed mock patient rooms to provide input on the best nursing and patient flow. At the ground-breaking ceremony, the CEO of the children's hospital made an announcement pointing us out in the crowd and thanking us for our contributions.

When a new building has reached the uppermost floor, it is customary to place a tree on the top as a symbol that the building has reached its highest elevation. The practice dates back to ancient Scandinavian times when a tree was placed atop a completed building to appease the tree-dwelling spirits that had been displaced at the building site. As usual, the children's hospital turned this into a mega media event. A small evergreen was hoisted by a crane to the roof of the building as the "topping off" tradition to the applause of all the employees and construction workers[82].

I later asked the CEO what would ultimately happen to the tree. "Not sure," he said brushing me off.

I suggested it would be a nice gesture to plant it on the perimeter of the building. I later found out it was donated instead to a nearby public park. As the building was being built, we held our first patient reunion for all the patients who had undergone fetal surgery at the new *fetal center*. The laser surgery for twin-twin transfusion had not always resulted in two surviving babies. My wife, now the lead nurse for our Center, had arranged a memorial service as part of the reunion. Patients who had lost one or both of their unborn babies were asked to write the names of their lost unborn children on a small rock. Karen asked if we could add these to the concrete floor of the new Fetal Center that was being built—a sort of time capsule of the lost souls from our early fetal surgeries.

"We don't honor dead babies here," she was told by a hospital administrator. "We only save babies here."

Things were changing in the Department of OB-GYN as well. The current Chairman was finally informed that he would be replaced by an acting Chair of OB-GYN. Despite ten years of service, the medical school decided there would be no celebration to honor the outgoing Chair. Our new acting Chair was nice enough but he had no experience in leading an academic department. I did my best to help recruit other MFM faculty.

In one case, James and I went to dinner with a local MFM to discuss referrals to the Fetal Center. She was a recent graduate from fellowship training and had been hired into private practice by a *neonatologist* (a high-risk pediatrician). This was an unusual business relationship. I assumed the *neonatologist* felt that this would increase the admissions (and revenue) for his neonatal intensive care unit. But things did not go well from the beginning. Office space was limited and the ultrasound equipment was suboptimal.

Karen leaned over to me during the dinner, "She can be easily recruited to our department."

Two days later we were working on a "napkin offer" over the phone. Dr. Stanford's partner caught wind of the change and let the neonatologist know. He fired her the next day.

She called me crying, "What am I to do? I have a house payment to make."

"Not to worry," I replied. "Will get you a letter and move up your start date."

I called the acting chair to let him know the situation. "Can you help me with a letter," he asked.

I wrote it that afternoon in between seeing patients in the ultrasound unit. Dr. Stanford was dutifully employed at the medical school the following week. She would soon set up a satellite MFM thriving office in a northern suburb of the city. It would ultimately be the model for the children's hospital to later develop a network of satellite MFM offices in the city.

Dr. Green had offered to be the *Acting Chairman* for two years, while the medical school searched for a full-time Chair. There was only one small problem. The previous divorce between the medical school and the adult teaching hospital had left the medical school in financial ruins. The school had tried to partner with a local well-known engineering university. They then entertained becoming a subsidiary of the main university whose namesake would then be used by the medical school. But both negotiations eventually failed when the magnitude of the financial deficits of the medical school was realized.

Recruiting a "franchise" Chairman of OB-GYN would require a financial commitment—promised funds to build a department. The children's hospital had done well in the 1980s. They had invested wisely and were rumored to have "a billion dollars" in their rainy-day account. And they were very good at raising donor funding. So, the Children's Hospital would be the primary source of funding for a new Chair. But they were not really that committed to overall women's health. They were really only interested in obstetrical patients. After all they would be the patients that would result in newborns being admitted to their nurseries and especially their intensive care units. But a good Chairman of a Department of OB-GYN has to give equal time to gynecology—well woman care, oncology, and infertility. Three rounds of prime candidates for the position were undertaken. But in all cases, the final negotiations ended when the primary emphasis on obstetrics was realized by the candidates. After two years, Dr. Green was under considerable pressure from his wife to give up the position as *acting chair*. After all the couple were in their 60's and loved to spend time at their second home in the mountains of Colorado.

The children's hospital asked Dr. Green to stay on. He agreed that if he could split his time between the city and his Colorado home at six-month intervals. He would make himself available through emails and phone calls when he was in Colorado. I suggested that perhaps we could form a "senior cabinet" to assist. We would act as advisors and be a "boots on the ground" team. Dr. Green agreed. When the six of us (appointed by Dr. Green) showed up for the first meeting, we were startled to see the retired original Chairman of the department attending. We were informed that the council would answer to him in Dr. Green's absence. The committee never met again. An email appeared in our inbox a week later. One of the members of the advisory group, the Director of the general OB-GYN Division, would be the Associate Chairman and would be in charge when Dr. Green was out of town.

Dr. Fitsimmons was the Chairman of Pediatrics for thirty-one years. He had acted as the CEO for the children's hospital in its early formative years. While still the Chairman, he had also served as the Dean of the medical school for seven years. He was a special individual. Even after he gave up the reins of administration of the Children's Hospital to a hospital administrator he had hand-picked, he was known for his morning rounds in the emergency room at 4 a.m. each day to check on the bed status of the hospital.

When James and I met with him to discuss our recruitment, we noted an extra young man sitting in the corner of the room.

"This is Tom, my hospital administrative intern," he informed us. "Anything you need to say to me, you can say in front of him. That's how I treat my administrative interns."

On one occasion, James and I were scheduled to meet with some high roller donors for the new woman's hospital. We were practicing our slide presentation on fetal surgery when Dr. Fitsimmons walked in. The forefinger of his right hand was notably wrapped with a bloody gauze.

"Caught the thing in the sliding door to the ER," he told us. "Didn't want to miss this meeting. I'll get the pediatric plastic guys to sew it up later."

"How does it feel?" I asked.

"Throbbing a bit," he responded.

The donors arrived and Fitsimmons made his excuses of a minor cut and then proceeded with the meeting. He returned to the ER two hours later for the suturing of his laceration.

Fitsimmons was probably too busy early in his career to take up routine exercise. But in his later years, he became an avid runner often holding meetings with key stakeholders during his morning jaunts. Soon after James and I had arrived to the medical center, he was diagnosed with small cell cancer of the lung and died only six months after his initial diagnosis. At his funeral, all three of his children delivered a eulogy. But it was his son, a construction supervisor, that delivered the most profound message. With Dr. Fitsimmons lying in state below the podium, he read a letter that his father had written only a few days earlier imploring the leaders of the medical school and the adult teaching hospital to put aside their differences and re-create their affiliation agreement. This would never come to pass.

Fitsimmons had always prided himself in having nurses and physicians in key leadership positions at the children's hospital. With his departure, the atmosphere at the hospital began to change to more of a corporate structure. The chief nursing officer had been recruited by Dr. Fitsimmons twenty years earlier. During our recruitment, she was one of the few leaders who understood what a fetal center would mean for admissions to the neonatal intensive care unit.

One day when she arrived at her office, a security officer was waiting to greet her. "Mam, please place your purse on the desk. I will escort you the parking lot," he said.

"But my keys are in my purse," she responded.

"That's Ok I'll bring them to you," he answered.

Mary later learned the hospital had decided to "go in a different direction." This maneuver later came to be known as *being walked*. I am sure that this method of termination is routinely practiced in corporate America. Basically, the employee is given no notice and computer access is denied on the day of the firing. My assumption is that administration feels that the disgruntled employee might use their access to corrupt or download computer files. In any event, it just doesn't sound like the way to treat an individual with long-standing loyalty.

And then there was the former NICU nurse who had shown great leadership potential at the children's hospital. A mother of two, she found the time to achieve a Masters of Business Administration. Fitsimmons had moved her into hospital administration and she was assigned to be our partner in creating the Fetal Center. Her initial meeting was with Karen, my wife. Karen had been our lead nurse for fetal surgery at the mid-Atlantic program, so we naturally made her part of the recruitment package for our new Fetal Center. She had arrived several weeks before James and I to get things organized.

I am sure this administrator ventured into the initial lunch meeting with the idea that we were "hiring the doctor's wife to arrange the flowers in the office." Three hours into the meeting, and two legal pads of notes later, she quickly realized that Karen would be an invaluable member of the team. Months after her boss was asked to leave the children's hospital, this nursing administrator was *walked* as well.

Dr. Fitsimmons had recruited two academic leaders in neonatal care from the East Coast—one would be the clinical Director of the NICU and the other would be the head of the Neonatology Division. A few months after Dr. Fitsimmons' untimely death, they were both *walked*. Rumor was that these two physicians (both tenured professors) had improved the quality of care in the NICU, resulting in a marked decrease in the overall length of hospital stay. This of course had affected the children's hospital's bottom line since NICU reimbursement was based on total number of hospital days that each infant remained hospitalized. The "old guard," a former neonatology fellow that previously trained at the institution, was recruited from a mid-Western hospital as their replacement.

Dr. Fugue, a former MFM fellow that I had helped train, would cross my academic path again.During his MFM fellowship, Dr. Fugue was predominantly interested in high-risk medical conditions in pregnant women. Arriving to the U.S. on a J-1 student visa, he had decided not to return to his native South Africa. At first his research efforts in women with pre-eclampsia were exemplary. He secured funding from the *Food and Drug Administration Orphan Drug Program* to study a new medication to prevent seizures in patients with high blood pressure. The study would eventually be published in the prestigious *New England Journal of Medicine*. At the conclusion of his fellowship training, there were two paths for individuals on a J-1 visa. One is to return to their native country for two years and then re-apply to return to the U.S. This policy was put in place to allow individuals to receive superior medical training in the American health system while not allowing the U.S. to be accused of being the "brain drain" for the world by keeping the most gifted physicians. Alternatively, one could stay in the U.S. after completing training by serving in an underserved medical area in the U.S. for two years. Dr. Fugue sought a third option. He had learned about a prominent immigration attorney from another South African physician who had been allowed to stay after completing his fellowship training under a "prominent academic achievement" premise. Fugue approached me for a letter of support since I was the Director of fellowship training at the time. We met and I agreed to the letter as long as he would commit to continue to pursue his fledging academic career.

"I will never go into private practice," he promised me.

I wrote a very strong letter and the attorney managed to get his visa changed. Fugue joined our Division as an attending for two years and then took a private practice position. It was lucrative enough that he eventually achieved a pilot's license and managed to purchase several planes.

Our paths would not cross again until I was at an international fetal surgery meeting in Aruba. Fugue was sitting in the lobby of the hotel talking to his wife on Skype. Karen pointed him out.

I went over to chat. "What brings you to this meeting?" I asked.

"Well, my partner and I are thinking about getting into fetal surgery and he told me this is the meeting I should attend," he responded.

Later I learned that the two of them had decided to become traveling fetal surgeons. They would travel to various institutions around the U.S. to do laser surgery for twin-twin transfusion. This did not make sense to me. James and I had learned from experience the difficulties with this procedure. The initial evaluation of the patient was important to decide if they were a candidate for the surgery with its inherent risk for premature delivery. In addition, a stable set of very special equipment and a trained operating room staff were paramount to the success of the procedure. After talking with several colleagues in the field, I authored an editorial in one of the major OB-GYN journals pointing out the detrimental issues with such an iterant fetal surgery practice. I would later find out that this editorial would probably have a profound effect on my future relationship with Fugue.

Fugue had applied for the position of Chair of OB-GYN in the department during the first round of interviews. He was not given serious consideration and was not invited for an interview. On the fourth round, however, the children's hospital was getting concerned about the lack of full-time leadership for the OB-GYN department. After all, the new Women's Hospital was due to open in few months and there would be the need for a new clinical Director. Fugue came for an interview. This would be a grand undertaking since it was the first time that a pediatric hospital was getting into the obstetrical business. Fugue did however boast a clinical professor appointment at a major medical school during his time in private practice. During the interview process, he was laudatory of our efforts to establish the Fetal Center over the previous five years.

"It would be a privilege to work with you guys," he told us.

James and I thought we had died and gone to heaven. A Chairman who understood what we did! This would mean real support for our efforts. This was a marked difference from the previous chair candidates that we had met. Most did not understand why we even had a fetal center at a children's hospital. We were therefore extremely supportive of Dr. Fugue's appointment as Chair. After a period of negotiations, he was offered the position of the Chairmanship of the OB-GYN department.

During the transition period, I had served as the MFM liaison on the Labor and Delivery operations committee. The committee consisted of administrators, nurses, midwives, and physicians. It met monthly to discuss policies and protocols involving patient care. An additional function of the committee was to decide on the implementation of new medications or devices that would be introduced to the obstetrical service. About a month after Fugue's appointment as Chair, I walked into a committee meeting to find a medical device company representative poised to make a presentation regarding a new OB device for the Labor and Delivery Unit. To say that this was out of the ordinary was an understatement. We had never had a representative of a device or pharmaceutical company attend the committee meeting. We wanted our discussions about the evaluation of new products for the OB service to be unencumbered by bias. *Postpartum hemorrhage* (massive bleeding after the delivery of a baby) is the number one cause of maternal death throughout the world. It accounts for more than one-fourth of all maternal deaths. The open site of the previous placenta implantation on the uterus continues to bleed, causing major blood loss. Various medications can be given to the pregnant patient to help the uterus to contract. When these are ineffective, a large balloon can be placed inside the uterus and filled with fluid. This compresses the vessels at the old placental site, stopping the bleeding. The most common device used for this is a *Bakri balloon*. We had begun to use the *Bakri balloon* in *atony* cases at my mid-Atlantic medical school. Upon returning to my former medical school, I had introduced the device to all of the obstetrical hospitals in the area. It was fairly cheap, easy to use, and quite effective. I am convinced that it saved several women from having to undergo a hysterectomy for their *postpartum hemorrhage*.

The unexpected guest at our committee meeting was there to promote a new uterine balloon for the treatment of *uterine atony*. She explained that the balloon had been designed by our new incoming Chairman and he would like to have it introduced into use on our Labor and Delivery Unit.

I inquired, "What is the cost of this new balloon?" It turned out it was three times more expensive than the *Bakri balloon*.

"And have there been any studies to compare it to the current balloon we are using?" I asked.

There were none. The rep stated that this was obviously a better device because it consisted of two balloons—one that entered the uterus and one that stayed in the vagina to keep the larger balloon in place in the uterus.

"And who holds the patent on this new device?" I asked.

"I believe it is Dr. Fugue," she replied.

I then moved that we excuse the rep from our committee meeting. After she left, I pointed out the conflict of interest that existed with the new Chairman's insistence on the use of a device where he had a clear financial incentive. I recommended that we not move forward with this device until we had the chance to undertake at least a comparative analysis of the new balloon with the one we were currently using.

About ten minutes after the meeting was over, I received a call on my cell phone from Fugue.

"Ken, I hear you were opposed to the use of the new balloon," he said.

"No", I responded. "I simply think we should evaluate this before we move forward. That has been the committee's usual practice. And besides, are you not concerned about a potential conflict of interest given that you hold the patent on the device?" I asked.

"Oh, I see," came the response.

In 2018, Dr. Jose Baselga resigned from his position at the Chief Medical Officer at the prestigious Sloan Kettering Cancer Institute[83]. During the previous four years, he had failed to disclose more than four million dollars of industry payments in more than 60% of the 180 articles he had authored. What made this case even more egregious was that he failed to disclose the industry payments in articles he published in the journal *Cancer Discovery*—a violation of the journal policy where he served as Editor-in-Chief. The core of this issue is the perception that such payments can influence the scientific integrity of the research. In other words—Is the quality of the research biased by funding by pharmaceutical support? The pharmaceutical and device industry now funds more than 60% of the biomedical research in the U.S. For this reason, academic researchers often work in conjunction with the industry to accelerate new discoveries in medicine. Such rare cases as that of Dr. Baselga have recently led to several changes in practice. All peer-review journals require a conflict of interest disclosure, whereby all authors must disclose industry payments for consulting and research as well as ownership in the companies. Agencies that certify continuing medical education events require a similar disclosure, with an initial slide added to the presentation to describe these disclosures to the audience. Medical schools now require that annual conflict of interest disclosures be filed by all faculty. Any new industry associations require prior approval by the Dean's office before implementation. Stock ownership in companies associated with ongoing research is forbidden by both the primary investigator as well as his/her first-degree relatives. Finally, the U.S. Congress included the *Sunshine Act* as an amendment as part of the *Affordable Healthcare Act* which passed in 2010[84]. Pharmaceutical companies, medical device companies, and medical supply companies that provide products covered by *Medicare, Medicaid,* or the *Children Health Insurance Program (CHIP)* are required to report monies paid to physicians to the *National Physician Payment Transparency Program.* The data can be viewed on a public website. Categories of payments include general, company ownership, and research funds.

The first day of Fugue's arrival as the new Chairman, I made a point to go by his office.

"Congrats on your appointment. I look forward to working with you," I said shaking his hand.

"Appreciate it," he responded. "You are the only one that has come by today."

Little did I realize, this would probably be the last time we would shake hands. Dr. Bogs, my mentor, once told me there were two types of leaders. The first would walk into the room where the candle of every faculty member was burning.

He would declare, "We need to get these candles burning more brightly." The second type of leader would walk into the same room. He would see all the individual candles burning and realize that they were stealing the light away from his candle. Several of these would need to be extinguished.

When James and I had arrived five years earlier, we did not challenge the leadership of the pediatric surgeons that had been appointed by the children's hospital as co-Directors of the fledging Fetal Center. Why should we? Although there had been some contentious times related to disagreements on how patients should be managed, we had grown to have mutual respect for one another. We all realized that we each brought a unique skill and perspective to the center.

It was time for an updated group photo for the Center. Fugue had announced that he would be doing fetal cases so he should be part of the photo. After waiting for him for about thirty minutes, the photographer decided to go ahead and take the picture of the four of us. Ten minutes later, our Chair showed up. We all had to pose again. This time Fugue positioned himself front and center of the group, arms folded. He was making a clear statement.

Later Fugue shared with James and me that as the new Chairman of OB-GYN, he was in essence the head of the Fetal Center. After all it would be housed in the new Women's Hospital and he would be the Chief of Obstetrics there. We shared with him that this was not a concept embraced by the two pediatric surgeons who had been appointed as co-Directors of the Center seven years earlier. Ultimately, this led to a contentious meeting with the group which included James, me, Fugue, the two pediatric surgeons, two pediatric hospital administrators, and the Director of the Division of Pediatric Surgery. At one point, Fugue told the Director of Pediatric Surgery that our department did not need his surgeons to run the Fetal Center. I was sitting at Fugue's right hand at the meeting.

"Can I try something?" I interjected. I went over to the dry erase board in the conference room and drew out a leadership flowchart. At the top of the chart, I put the Chairman of OB-GYN, the next level would be two co-Directors—one from MFM and one from pediatric surgery. The final level would consist of an executive committee of representatives of other key specialties. Dr. James agreed that this represented a reasonable compromise for a leadership model. He then left the room briefly to answer a page. Fugue rejected the proposal and the meeting disbanded soon thereafter. The next day, my secretary brought me a typed letter from Fugue. The letter was a reprimand for my not supporting his leadership position at the previous day's meeting.

Until then, I interpreted these events as a bump in the road. Surely this was the inexperience of a new Chairman having to evolve his leadership style. Our Fetal Center was now known in national academic circles. We had recruited a fellow for training and he had been prolific, presenting his research at national and international meetings and in peer-review publications.

An NIH-funded trial had just been completed that demonstrated that fetal surgery for spina bifida could have a dramatic impact on the outcome of these children after birth[85]. Since I had been involved in performing ten cases prior to the initialization of the trial, I proposed that I be the point person for bringing the surgery to our center. I arranged visits to two of the institutions that had participated in the trial—one was where I had undertaken my OB-GYN residency. The pediatric neurosurgeon there was the first in the world to perform the procedure. Having done almost 175 cases before the trial had begun, he clearly had the most experience in the technique of fetal repair of spina bifida. He agreed to come to our institution as part of their team to assist us with our first case. I thought this would be a real feather in the cap of our Fetal Center.

I called Fugue just a few minutes after my phone call with the pediatric neurosurgeon to share the news. He was elated. Later that day, Fugue was slated to give grand rounds for the Department of Pediatrics to share his vision for the Department of OB-GYN. He arrived just as the lecture was scheduled to begin and there was a computer malfunction so he was unable to start with his Power

Point presentation. While the IT folks were addressing the problem, he began to talk extemporaneously. James and I were attending the grand rounds, seated at the top of the auditorium. Fugue began by singing the accolades of the Fetal Center and how it was nationally recognized. He intended to make it bigger and better. Then he announced that just that day, we had managed to invite a prominent pediatric neurosurgeon from another institution to assist with our first open fetal surgery case for the in- utero repair of spina bifida. I watched the Chief of Cardiovascular Surgery and the Chief of Pediatric Neurosurgery seated in the front row of the auditorium shift uneasily in their seats.

I looked at James. "Can you believe he just said that?" I asked. "I just told him about my call an hour ago."

"Let's see their reaction at the end of this lecture," he responded.

Forty-five minutes later at the end of the lecture and the usual applause, the two heads of surgery were the first out of their chairs to talk with Fugue.

An hour later, I received an urgent phone call from him.

"How could you do this to me?" he asked.

"Do what?" I asked.

"You didn't talk to either the Chief of Surgery or the Chief of Pediatric Neurosurgery about the visiting pediatric neurosurgeon coming to assist in a fetal surgery?" he asked.

"That would be difficult," I responded. "I had just gotten off the phone with him an hour earlier. And since they both would have to agree to give him temporary surgical privileges at our hospital, my plan was to check in with them later."

"Well, I will be the one giving out surgical temporary privileges at the new Women's Hospital anyway so I don't need their permission," he replied.

A week later we were all in Fugue's office for a meeting—Fugue, myself, the head of pediatric neurosurgery, and his junior neurosurgeon. Another contentious meeting ensued. The head of pediatric neurosurgery stated that his surgeons were quite skilled and there was no need for "instruction" by a neurosurgeon from another institution. After all they had experience in performing spina bifida repairs in premature infants and fetal surgery could not be any more challenging than that.

Fugue responded, "I believe it would be unethical to proceed with this program without taking advantage of the experience of a neurosurgeon that has performed hundreds of these cases."

The meeting ended with no final agreement on the future course of action.

At the end of the meeting, Fugue looked at me. "How do you think that went?" he asked.

I knew better but to simply agree. "I think you held your ground," I responded.

A year later, the first in utero repair would be performed at the children's hospital without the expertise of a visiting pediatric neurosurgeon.

When we designed the Fetal Center area in the new women's hospital, our group lobbied hard to have adjoining offices to our clinical space. We proposed that our academic offices could be utilized for patient counseling as well, thus creating a collaborative atmosphere for the physicians. This was a radical concept for the children's hospital. Academic physicians were routinely assigned office space in a separate building from clinical space. Small consult rooms were usually located in the clinical space to meet with patients and their families. We finally convinced the hospital administration to recon-sider the concept. The offices of two MFM's, two pediatric surgeons, a radiologist, and a pediatric cardiologist were all designed in one office suite next to the ultrasound rooms. Eventually as the building neared completion, we were taken on a tour of the space and shown carpet and wallpaper swatches to pick out colors.

One of our intake coordinators at our Fetal Center was sched-uled to get married a week later. Having become close to the family, Karen and I were invited to the rehearsal dinner and wedding which took place in another city. James gave me a call just before the rehearsal dinner was scheduled to start on Friday evening.

"A new development," he said. "Fugue has decided to turn our office space into clinic space so the MFM Division can see private patients."

Our pediatric surgery colleagues were furious. Up until now the four main physicians that saw patients in the center had been housed in two separate buildings. Patients had to be escorted across a skybridge to be seen by all members of the group. Separate meet-ings had to be held weekly to plan the patient's care. A common office space in the women's hospital would allow for essential collaboration.

On Monday, an emergency meeting of the physician leadership of the Fetal Center took place. The two pediatric surgery co-Directors suggested that the four of us meet with children's hospital adminis-tration to voice our disapproval with Fugue's plan. James and I said we could not participate given the current tension with our Chair. The co-Directors went ahead with the meeting. In the interim, we met with Fugue to explain that although he felt that his new position as Chair allowed him to be in control of the Fetal Center, the two pediatric surgeons did not work for him as they answered to the Chair of Surgery. surgeons did not work for him as they answered to the Chair of Surgery. It was their impression that they were still the co-Directors of the center.

I was about to leave my office later that day when my pager went off. I was being summoned to the chair's office. *What now?* I thought.

The hospital administration had shared the pediatric co-Directors' dissatisfaction with the recent decision regarding the office space. Fugue was furious with James and me.

"Why had you not warned me of this?" he admonished us.

We tried to point out that we had predicted this from our previous conversations but he would not let us speak at the meeting. The next day we both received letters of reprimand (my second).

I decided that things were looking bleak for my staying at this institution. I met with the human resources department at the medical school to ask about my rights as a tenured professor.

"Well, since we are a private medical school, a third letter of reprimand could result in a non-renewal of your contract at the end of the academic year," I was told.

Our initial five-year contract was over and the medical school had begun to issue annual contracts at the start of each academic year. I decided to meet with Fugue to see if I could repair the damage. He came to my office.

"I am not sure how to start, but I feel that you believe that James and I have not been supportive of your leadership. After two letters of reprimand, I feel like I have a target on my back. This has become an uncomfortable place for me to work. I would like to ask if we could put these previous experiences behind us and start with a fresh slate."

"I can't do that," he told me.

"Well if you want me to leave, I'll start looking but please do not put me on the street. I have kids in college and a house payment to make."

He promised me that he would not.

James called me to his office the next day. Fugue had met with him to discuss my leaving. He offered for him to stay to run the Fetal Center. What Fugue had not counted on was a long-standing comradery between James and me. We had always aspired to work together and I had finally made this happen at two different institutions. More importantly we had both come to realize our dream of developing a niche in fetal medicine.

I arranged a meeting with the former Director of Neonatology at the children's hospital who had been previously *walked* from his job. He had recovered well—he was now the Chairman of Pediatrics at the other medical school in our city. Mary, the former Director of Nursing at the children's hospital who had also been *walked*, was now the Chief Operating Officer of the children's hospital down the street. A meeting between the two of us was scheduled. When I walked into the restaurant, I was greeted by Mary and another physician who I hardly knew. He'd been recruited to the OB-GYN department of the nearby medical school to maintain their NIH maternal network research unit.

"I am a bit confused," I said. "I thought I was meeting with Mary."

Mary spoke up. "Things are about to change in the Department. The current Chair will be asked to step down soon and we will have a new acting Chair. She has not been told yet, so mum is the word."

I was starting to have flashbacks again!

"What I need from you is some information on the patient numbers from the Fetal Center so I can sell this to the Dean and the hospital," Mary told me.

I reached into my pocket and pulled out the latest copy of our *dashboard* (an analysis of patient numbers and their associated revenue).

"Exactly what I needed," she said.

James had decided to take a week of vacation during this time to figure out where he was headed in his career.

The night he returned, I gave him a call. "I have something brewing for the two of us," I told him. "Stay tuned."

A few days later, Mary, the acting Chair of the new OB-GYN department and the Dean of the medical school met with James and me at my house. Although our city is the fourth largest in the U.S., folks have a tendency not to roam very far. We could not afford for this group to be seen at a local restaurant. Negotiations were quick— we would be named as co-Directors of the fetal center with the pediatric surgeon who was already there attempting to get a fetal center started. Karen, my wife, would be our lead nurse and we would hire two research personnel. Another meeting occurred a few nights later with the Chairman of Pediatric Surgery and his junior faculty—we convinced them that we could be collaborative to build a world-class center. We signed contract letters a few days later.

Two weeks later, I wrote letters of resignation for the James and myself, placed them in sealed envelopes, and delivered them to Dr. Fugue's office. We decided given the current state of affairs that we would only give a two-week notice. I received a phone call at around 10 a.m. It was Fugue.

"I need to meet with you as soon as possible in my office," he said.

"I really cannot meet right now," I replied. "This is a very emotional day for me."

James called me about an hour later. He was in the ultrasound unit seeing patients for the Fetal Center that day.

"What gives? I have been locked out of my EMR?" he asked.

I checked my email. It was no longer active.

I called him back. "I guess they have locked both of us out of all computer programs," I said.

"Well, I thought it might go this way so I have been taking home all the stuff out of my office over the course of this week," James said.

Another call from the Chairman's office. It was the departmental administrator.

"I am headed over to get your keys and your ID badge," she said.

Not anticipating this series of events, I had not even begun to pack up my office. I started to put books and family photos in wire baskets to take to my car. The word rapidly spread throughout the building. Sonographers and genetic counselors that worked with us appeared at my office door to help. Many were in tears.

The departmental administrator also appeared at my door. "Your badge, please," she said. "And don't worry about packing up your office, we can take care of this for you."

"Not going to happen," I responded. "I am a tenured professor. The only way you will *walk* me is to bring hospital security here."

The office was bare thirty minutes later. Everything had been thrown haphazardly into my car. I left my keys and my ID badge on my desk. Despite previous promises, we were on the street without a job or health insurance for our families.

We called the Dean at our new medical school the next day to explain the situation. He agreed to move up our start date. I heard later that our leaving had sent reverberations throughout the medical school of our former employment. A new policy was adopted that faculty would be required to give a three-month notice before their departure or they would forfeit their matched retirement funds from the school. I also later learned that James' outstanding medical records from his last day were signed by another physician so that billing could be undertaken. This physician did not see these patients.

Medical schools once patterned themselves like their university counterparts. But these events had taught me that a new corporate-like culture had now become the norm at medical schools. Physicians are often salaried by medical schools, although some schools use incentive pay generated from patient care activities as part of the salary structure. Yet the intellectual property of full-time faculty is often deemed the property of the medical school. Take patents for example. Most schools will share any financial return on any newly patented invention with a faculty. The school pays the initial legal expenses to file the patent and then any profits from a subsequent start-up company or the sale of a patent are split 50:50 once the initial expenses have been covered. This seems relatively fair to the physician. However, the terms of this agreement can even extend to work performed during a physician's own personal time.

Research materials are even more problematic when a physician leaves a school. Are the samples that they have collected over many years for a particular research project the property of the school or the property of the investigator? Given that the samples were collected for a specific purpose, it would make sense that the physician would be allowed to move the samples to a new institution to continue their research. This not always the case.

We had amassed a database of over 300 patients that had undergone laser surgery for twin-twin transfusion since our Fetal Center had started. The data collection had been approved by the medical school's investigation review board and the patients had all signed consents. These were not medical records but various data points that we had collected to study any factors that might predict the success of the surgery. We had developed the database and personally entered the data ourselves. So, on the day we left, thinking this was *our data,* we took copies of the database and the patient consents. What ensued over the next several days were threats from the children's hospital and the medical school attorneys regarding the *theft* of confidential patient data.

The *Health Care Portability and Accountability Act (HIPPA)* was passed by the Congress in 1996 and signed by President Clinton[86]. The law covered several facets of healthcare insurance including allowing patients to transfer their coverage when they changed employment and the establishment of medical savings accounts. The main tenet however of *HIPPA* was to address the confidentially of patients' private information (so-called *protected health information or PHI*). A later update to the legislation created significant civil and criminal penalties for violation of *HIPPA*. If an individual "unknowingly" discloses *PHI*, civil fines ranging from $100 to $50,000 can be levied. A "knowing" disclosure can result in criminal charges with a fine of $50,000 and one year in prison. The sale of *PHI* can result in criminal charges with a fine of $250,000 and up to ten years in prison.

The attorneys at our new medical school advised us based on the potential for a *HIPPA* violation that we should return the database and patient consent documents. Negotiations between the deans of the two medical schools transpired. A recent exodus of transplant surgeons across the neighboring medical schools had resulted in a similar dispute regarding a database and our new dean had decided to release the data to his former faculty. We expected the same. The final agreement was to purge the database of all *PHI* and release only the surgical data points by case number. This *de-identified data* is how most clinical research is done today when large databases of patient information are shared. Fugue reviewed the database and decided that there were too many missing data points invalidating the data-set. He never released the data.

Needless to say, the children's hospital that we recently left was not thrilled with having a competitive fetal center just blocks down the street. They realized that the close relationships we had formed with referring MFM's over the previous five years would result in a competitive edge over the inexperienced faculty at their institution. Around that time, Karen had suggested that we simplify the name of our new Fetal Center to match the URL on their center website. This included the name of the state where the center was located. After all, the URL had been purchased years earlier. The hospital attorney advised us to file a copyright on the name as well.

Our previous institution discovered the copyright application and filed an injunction to cease and desist. After all, they proposed the name of the new center might lead to confusion by patients and physicians since our name mirrored part of the name of their hospital. A lawsuit ensued and depositions were taken. During the course of these, it was discovered that the marketing team had sent out letters to our referring physicians announcing our new affiliation. Karen had told them to purchase a mailing list from our national MFM organi-zation but an inexperienced member of the marketing team at our new hospital had instead decided to use a copy of the spreadsheet of names of referring physicians from our former center. Again, it came down to who owned this information. In the end, our new institution decided it was not worth the cost of the legal fees to contest the matter. Our center name was changed to *The Fetal Center*.

19

The Doctor Is a Patient

I had never really been sick before in my life. I remember being in bed for a week with the flu several years earlier. The muscle aches and high fever made it feel like someone had beaten me with a wooden bat. A year later, our hospital began to require that all physicians would need to be immunized with the annual flu vaccine. This was of course more for the protection of the patients than the institution looking out for its healthcare work force. In 2011, our state passed legislation requiring every licensed hospital to develop a policy for mandating and recording required vaccinations and testing for all employees, physicians, and volunteers. For the pediatric hospital where I worked this included documentation of immunity to rubella, measles, mumps, and chickenpox as well as a current immunization record of diphtheria and whooping cough. All hospitals required annual tuberculosis skin testing for infection as well as annual influenza vaccines. If a healthcare worker refuses the influenza vaccine (allergy to eggs or just plain doesn't believe in it), then the policy mandated the individual must wear a surgical mask when on the hospital premises between Dec 1st and March 30th.

It was Christmas break and I had the week off. I began to develop generalized body aches and a high fever. I had received the required influenza vaccine a few months earlier but invariably the chance of still getting the flu is about 10%–20%. The influenza virus is one of the smartest viruses that infect mankind. It has been responsible for many pandemics—a rapid worldwide spread of the virus with its associated deaths. Millions of individuals have died in these pandemics—mostly the very young, the very old, and others with chronic medical conditions. The most devastating of these occurred in 1918 near the end of World War I[87]. More than fifty million people died—more than three times the number of lives lost in the war. The influenza virus mutates—it changes two different proteins on the outside of the viral particle almost yearly. This confuses the human immune system. Even though one may have developed immunity to last year's strain of virus, this mutated virus is almost like seeing a whole new insult to the immune system. So we have to get a new vaccine every year.

The *World Health Organization (WHO)* maintains influenza surveillance centers in six different units located in Atlanta, Melbourne, London, Tokyo, Beijing, and Koltsovo[88]. A meeting is held each February to make a recommendation on the most likely three or four strains of the flu virus that will appear in the next season (another meeting is held in September to make recommendations for a Southern Hemisphere vaccine since their winter months are opposite to those in the Northern Hemisphere). The *FDA* has the final say as to what strains will be in the annual influenza vaccine in the United States. So basically, the experts make an educated guess, and sometimes they get it wrong.

This was the case the year I came down with my fever. With high fevers and muscle aches, I reasoned it must be the flu. I called one of my colleagues to phone in a prescription to a local pharmacy for *oseltamivir* (*Tamiflu®*). The medication is not a cure—it basically slows the spread of the virus and decreases the symptoms by only one to two days. A week later I was not getting better. Patients that are ill can seldom make rational decisions about their care. This holds true for physicians as well. Nurses will tell you we make the worse patients. Individuals who study this phenomenon have labeled it *childhood regression*—we just want someone else to take care of us and make all the decisions. My wife, not ever used to seeing me very ill for this length of time, put on her nursing cap. She took me to an urgent care clinic. A nasal swab for the flu virus was negative. A chest X-ray showed no signs of pneumonia. The ER doc on duty suggested I go to the hospital emergency room if I did not improve in forty-eight hours.

Karen took me the emergency room twenty-four hours later. During the holidays, we had been staying on our property about twenty miles outside of our state's capital. The hospital where we went was deemed the medical center for the city, although it was not associated with a medical school. This would come some years later when the taxpayers of the city decided it was high time for the state capital to have its own medical school. At the hospital ER, the attending physician took my history and examined me. He could find no clear source of infection. My white blood cell count was elevated as were my liver tests. He felt the latter could have been related to the ibuprofen I was taking every six hours to keep my fever down. A chest X-ray and CT scan of my abdomen did not reveal any clues. He consulted with an infectious disease expert by phone who agreed to see me in the office the following morning.

Karen drove me to the office appointment the next day. Jack Binder was of a similar age as myself. I would later determine that he was "old school." He believed in starting with a complete history and physical. A review of my history alone took thirty minutes.

"When did my fever start?" he began with the inquiry. "What had I taken? Who was sick at home? Did any of my patients or their fetuses have a rare infection that might have been transmitted to me? Did I remember any tick bites? What kind of animals did I encounter on my property?"

I related that I had trapped some wild hogs on the property that were becoming a nuisance when they were rooting up all the gardens. I had helped one of the workers butcher them. Could this be the source? Feral hogs carry strange bacterial disease like tularemia and brucellosis. I had no domesticated animals.

"Were there any chicken farms nearby?" he continued. Salmonella and avian flu can be transmitted to humans. Dr. Binder told me about a patient he had seen previously who had become ill with a fever. He had acquired an air-borne bacteria from a chicken farm that was downwind of his ranch. None of these ideas seemed to be the culprit but a series of blood tests would be necessary to be sure. Nothing showed up on my physical examination.

At this point, Binder suggested that we order the tests, then I could return to see him later in the week. Karen jumped in as my advocate.

"I have been married to this man for thirty years. He is never sick. I want him admitted to the hospital," she insisted.

Jack relented. There were no beds that were available yet from the day's discharges. The admitting office said they would call us as soon as one was vacant. Being an hour drive back to the property, we decided to get a milkshake and wait for the call. I normally love milkshakes—strawberry is my favorite flavor. But on this day, I only finished about a quarter of the drink. In fact, I had not felt like eating much for the past two weeks—and I had lost almost ten pounds. Two hours later, we received a call that a room was ready. Once I was admitted, there were a whole series of blood tests that were drawn and an IV was started to give me some fluids.

Bender came by later that evening. We would not start any antibiotics until my fever had returned and he could draw some special lab tests called *blood cultures* to see if there were any specific bacteria in my blood stream. My temperature went up to 104 that night. The blood cultures were drawn and the Tylenol brought my temperature down nicely. Jack came by the next morning.

"Let's try to get one more set of *blood cultures* today if you have a fever and then we will start some general antibiotics," he said. I'm going to order a *CT* scan of the chest today as well."

Karen came by later that morning. I told her I did not want her to stay in the hospital—I would be fine. That second early evening, there was a knock at my door. A young physician entered and introduced herself as the *hospitalist* on call. She asked a few questions about my illness and said she was available through the night if anything changed. Later that evening my temperature again became elevated to 102. Blood cultures were drawn and I was given Tylenol. An hour later, the nurse arrived with a bag of IV fluids that appeared to be labeled as if they contained a medication.

"Hate to be a pest. Can you tell me what that is in the bag?" I asked.

"Yes, the hospitalist ordered an antibiotic for your fever," she replied.

"Can we hold on that?" I said. "I think Dr. Bender wants to see the results of the first blood culture before he puts me on antibiotics. Can you give him a call?"

She said that she would. She never returned that night to administer the antibiotics.

The next morning Jack came by on rounds.

"I apologize for what transpired last night," he said. "These *hospitalists* work a couple of shifts per week and rarely know what is going on with the patients. The chest CT only showed a little fluid outside of your lungs. No real source of infection. We have negative blood cultures so far. I am going to start you on some broad-spectrum antibiotics that should cover most bugs."

That early evening, a new *hospitalist* stopped by. She asked me the same questions about my history all over again. I tried to be a good patient and recounted my story yet another time knowing full well that it would not change my care. She did however listen to my heart and lungs with her stethoscope; something the previous *hospitalist* had not done. An orderly appeared at my door the next morning at around 7 a.m..

"Time for your echo," he said.

"Ok, I didn't know I was getting one of these," I replied. About that time, Bender appeared for morning rounds.

"Where are you taking him?" he inquired.

"To get an *echocardiogram*," responded the orderly.

"And who in the blazes ordered that?" he asked.

"Not sure, doc. Just move patients when I am told," he replied.

Jack left to review the chart and returned a few minutes later. "I cancelled the order," he told me. "Seems the *hospitalists* have struck again. You do not have *bacterial endocarditis* (an infection of the heart valves of the heart)! There is no reason to get the echo."

I was once a visiting professor at a medical school and after I gave grand rounds, I was asked to meet with the OB-GYN residents. It is customary at these meetings to pick another medical topic to discuss with the residents. "Let's forego a medical topic and talk about future careers in medicine," I said. "Now let me propose that I will pay each of you $150,000 a year. You will get three weeks of vacation and two weeks leave for educational meetings. I will need six of you to provide twenty-four hours-a-day, seven days-a-week coverage of my Labor and Delivery Unit. You will need to work three twelve-hour shifts each week. Some will be day shifts and some will be night shifts. Cross-coverage for holidays and pregnancy leave will be worked out among the group. How many of you want to work for me?" Of the twenty residents at the meeting, twelve hands went up. The career choice I was describing was that of a *hospitalist*.

In the past, the typical OB-GYN in private practice would make rounds at the hospital each morning, head over to their office by 9 a.m., see forty patients or so during the course of the day, and then make evening rounds at 6 p.m. Sometimes they would be called to deliver a patient in the middle of the day. This would result in a two to three hour increased wait time for the patients at their office that were previously scheduled.

The OB would usually apologize to his waiting patients, "I have to go deliver a baby. Be right back." This typically appeased them since they would want the same treatment when they are about to deliver.

The physician would share night and weekend calls with other members of the group practice so that they may need to sleep at the hospital every third or fourth night if one of the group's patients was in labor. The next day after call, they would repeat the same office schedule even though they may not have slept much the previous night. Sleep deprivation of less than five hours per night has been associated with an increased risk for various chronic diseases as well as increased mortality[89]. This hectic schedule is not only a contributor to poor health for the physicians but the patients also do not always receive optimal care. Studies have shown that this model of private practice resulted in the peak times of the day when C-sections are performed to be 7 a.m. and 5 p.m. Scheduled C-sections are usually done in the morning before clinics start. Evening C-sections are usually done after clinic hours if the patient had not made good progress in labor during the day[90]. After all, the tired OB-GYN would like to see his family at some point in the evening. Pregnant patients that had been previously delivered by C-section for such indications as breech presentation can undergo a safe vaginal delivery or trial of labor (TOL) in most cases. If successful the procedure is called a *Vaginal Birth After Cesarean Section (VBAC)*. The chance for a vaginal birth may be as high as 86% if the patient has a history of a previous vaginal birth[91]. If the incision on the uterus from the previous C-section is transverse, the risk for rupture of the uterine scar in labor is less than 1%. However, in the case of a rupture, the fetus can develop a slow heart rate due to the lack of oxygen. An emergency C-section must be performed in under fifteen minutes. For this reason, physicians with a busy practice are reluctant to take on this responsibility and offer a *TOL* to their patients. In fact, some hospitals have policies in place on how far away the physician can be if they are allowing one of their patients to attempt a *TOL*.

The term *hospitalist* first appeared in the medical literature in 1996[92]. Primarily confined to the specialty of internal medicine for many years, the role has now entered the field of obstetrics. An even newer role is that of the *nocturnalist*—an obstetrician who covers Labor and Delivery only during the evening shift from Sunday night through Thursday night. This role has been developed to parallel that of the night float rotation that was introduced in most OB-GYN residency training programs to allow for adherence to the *ACGME* duty hour requirements. There are clear advantages to a *hospitalist* model. Physicians are more likely to get proper rest. Patients benefit from the constant presence of a physician who is immediately available for emergencies. This allows for more cases of *TOL* and less "end of the day" C-sections.

But there are clear disadvantages. Continuity of care (much like in my case) is interrupted and there is the chance for errors during handoffs much like what occurs with the night float system in residency training. The current model of reimbursement for obstetrical care pays a global fee to the OB-GYN physician—fourteen prenatal visits, a delivery, and a postpartum visit. Since the delivery fee comprises almost 60% of the global reimbursement, private OB-GYN's are reluctant to allow the *hospitalist* to bill for their deliveries. This has led most hospitals to pay the salaries of the *hospitalists*. Will this continue in the face of rising hospital costs in the future or will the model of obstetrical care become segmented into outpatient and inpatient charges? More importantly, will patients accept a physician unknown to them as their delivering obstetrician. My prediction is that they will have little choice in the near future. And then who will undertake the gynecologic surgeries that women will need? Will this be another subset of OB-GYNs? It does not take long to realize that we will need more OB-GYN physicians in this changing model. Will other allied healthcare professionals such as physician associates, nurse practitioners, and midwives enter the model to allow the system to be more cost-effective? I suspect this will be the case.

Dr. Bender proceeded to update me on the tests he had ordered since my admission to the hospital.

"To be honest, I am not sure what you have," he said. "All the cultures are negative. The serologic tests for all the rare infections have returned negative—it's not the chickens or the hogs. You don't have leukemia or multiple myeloma. Let's give the antibiotics a few more days and see if you respond."

Over the next forty-eight hours, I began a game with the evening shift of nurses. I knew when I was spiking a fever and I had gotten pretty good at determining how high it was. I would guess and then they would take my temperature. Little changed. Markers for inflammation continued to be elevated on daily blood checks—my *white blood cell count, sedimentation rate, and C-reactive protein*.

Karen was becoming frantic with the lack of a diagnosis. She had confronted Bender on the lack of a progress.

"Maybe you should take him to a real medical center," he replied.

"But this hospital has *medical center* in its name, doesn't it?" she inquired. At that point she began to make arrangements to take me back to the major medical center where I worked three hours away. She even called the CEO of my hospital and asked if they could arrange for a helicopter transport. They said they would.

The next day, Jack arrived for morning rounds and said that he had talked with one of his *rheumatology* colleagues about my case (*rheumatologists* care for patients with various forms of arthritis and autoimmune diseases like *lupus* and *rheumatoid arthritis*). They had reviewed the lab values and my clinical course. His colleague had suggested a diagnosis of *Still's disease*.

Still's disease is a rare autoimmune disease occurring in only in two individuals in one million. Its peak age at onset is thirt-six years; it is even rarer in patients over fifty years of age like myself[93]. *Still's* is in the family of autoimmune diseases like rheumatoid arthritis and can present with fever, arthritis, and muscle aches. A case is often presented for management on the internal medicine written boards so most internists know of the disease but few ever see a patient with it—especially at my age. Jack gave me the print out from *UpTo-Date*—an online reference written by experts in many fields. He said the rheumatologist would be by later but that we would try a course of high-dose intravenous steroids to see if my fever would respond.

The rheumatologist came by later that afternoon and went over the plan. He agreed with Jack that *Still's* was the likely diagnosis even though I did not have all of the classic clinical symptoms. He would order a few more lab tests to confirm that this was not another auto-immune disease, but there was no real diagnostic test for *Still's*. We would have to see how I responded to the intravenous steroids.

The steroids were started at around 4 p.m. I fully expected my fever would spike a few hours later like it had been doing for the last three weeks. I did run a low-grade fever later that night to about 100 degrees. And then I began to sweat profusely! It was almost like my body wanted to release all the toxins that had accumulated over the past few weeks all at one time. In fact, I perspired so much that night, that the nurses had to change my gown and bedsheet three times! I was sent home the next day on steroids by mouth.

I saw the rheumatologist in his office the next day and he made a referral to the head of the rheumatology division at my medical school in my hometown. Steroids are an interesting medication. Our body releases its own steroids in times of stress from two small glands located on the top of each kidney (the *adrenal glands*). But oral steroids in high doses produce levels of stress hormone that are much higher than usual. They increase your appetite, interrupt sleep, and cause mood swings. Long-term use of steroids can cause excessive hair growth (*hirsutism*), acne, bone thinning (*osteoporosis*), and the infamous *buffalo hump* (a collection of fat between the shoulder blades near the back of the neck). Needless to say, I wanted off the steroids. They gave me *urinary frequency* (is there a bathroom nearby?) and knee pain.

I met my new *rheumatologist* a week later. Dr. Reeves was about my age and a big conversationalist. He was well-published, NIH grant-funded, and held an international reputation in the world of *rheumatology*. I was lucky to become one of his patients as he had decided to limit his practice to just a few of his long-standing patients. We hit it off at the first visit often sharing stories of unusual patients and lamenting how medicine had changed over the course of our careers.

Reeves hated steroids—"Bad for you. Can give you hip fractures after only a few short months," he said. "Let's wean you off these in the next few weeks and try you on an old fallback medicine called *methotrexate.*"

I agreed. *Methotrexate* was introduced in 1948 as chemotherapy for leukemia. Later it became the mainstay for therapy for rheumatoid arthritis. It is cheap—about sixty dollars a month. It was well tolerated except for its occasional association with liver damage.

"We will follow blood work every few months, but I am more interested in how you are feeling," he said. I would not be able to drink alcohol on the methotrexate—not a problem since I routinely volunteered to be the designated driver even for my wife. Off steroids I realized that my major symptoms were early evening fatigue, an inflammation in my throat that caused me to cough, and a low-grade fever. My labs, particularly my *C-reactive protein (CRP)*, indicated a continued low grade of inflammation. A chronic state of inflammation is now considered a risk factor for the development of heart disease. So, Reeves and I agreed that we would like to see me get to a normal *CRP* level.

When I finally returned to work, I learned that one of the sonographers at our office had battled *Still's disease* since she was in college.

"You're so lucky," she informed me. "They diagnosed you quickly. It took them years to figure out what I had. There were days when I could not crawl out of my bed."

At an incidence of two people per one million population, we joked that we represented 16% of the six million inhabitants of our city who had *Still's disease*. Of course, the chance that two individuals with *Still's disease* would work in the same office was one in 250 billion! Jennie and I would later share trade secrets about our therapies. She had been on methotrexate for many years. When she was later considering pregnancy, she had been switched to a new medication called *anikara* long before I would eventually learn about this drug.

Every one of my repeat blood tests for *CRP* would remain elevated and I still did not feel like my old self. We decided to increase the methotrexate over the usual upper limits of the recommended dose. After all I was not a drinker. Still the *CRP* would not come down and my liver tests rose to twice the normal levels. Time for a switch.

In general, insurance companies would like physicians to start with the cheapest of proven therapies for a condition before moving to more expensive ones. This is not always the case. Patients will often see a television advertisement for an exciting new drug and ask their physicians to prescribe it. "Will my insurance cover this?" is the usual question. If the physician says yes, then they want to please (and keep) their patient, so they acquiesce. Dr. Reeves agreed with me that we should set the example and start with the cheapest medication, but in this case, it was not achieving our goal. He recommended moving to *anikara,* a monoclonal antibody that has to be injected under the skin on a daily basis.

Monoclonal antibodies are the latest breakthrough in the world of cancer and autoimmune diseases. Courtesy of the incredible basic science research that has occurred in our country, we now have a growing understanding of how our immune system works and in the case of cancer and autoimmune disease—and how it fails us. Human antibodies can now be manufactured in the cell lines of hamster ovaries and tailored to block certain targets on our cells called *receptors.* In my case, *anikara* would block the receptor for *inter-leukin-1 (IL-1)*—a chemical (also called a *cytokine*) in my body that was elevated due to my *Still's disease.*

This would not be a cheap medication—about $3,000 each month. My medical insurance through my medical school would cover the costs except for a twenty-dollar monthly co-pay. This would result in a change in my lifestyle. Every day I would need to awaken, warm the syringe from the refrigerator, and inject myself in my lower abdomen much like a diabetic gives themselves insulin. In the beginning, as predicted by the package insert, I would get itchy whelps every place I injected. And then I would have to remember to "rotate" the injection sites each day so as to not give the medication in the same location.

During the first few months, I would put ice on the spot for about a minute to numb the area. After about six months, I decided to simply plunge the needle in quickly. Because *Anikara (Kinerat®)* causes a significant suppression of the immune system, I would have to be checked for tuberculosis with a blood test every year.

I could not take any vaccines that contained a live virus. On one occasion, I was invited to consult with a teaching obstetrical hospital in Ethiopia. I had always dreamed of "giving back" later in my academic career by helping to improve obstetrical care in developing countries. But an outbreak of yellow fever in Ethiopia would mean I would be required to be vaccinated for this disease. The yellow fever vaccine is a live virus—so this would not be possible. I would have to decline the invitation.

Finally, there was the travel issue. I am often invited in my role as an academician to give lectures at other universities. This means that the Transportation Security Administration (TSA) folks would become my friends. I purchased a special medication bag from Amazon that contained a sealed plastic block that could be frozen. This would keep the syringes of medication cold for about eight hours. The bag contained a small battery and a thermometer to tell you the temperature inside the bag. On my very first run through the TSA line at the airport I heard, "bag check." A TSA agent asked me if this was my bag and would I step over to the side for a special inspection. He proceeded to pull up the image from the X-ray machine.

"What's in the bag?" he asked.

"My medication. It has needles but they are capped," I responded. He unzipped the small canvas bag to review its contents.

"See here this looks like C-4, a block of plastic explosive," he said. "And that looks like a battery" and then pointing to the thermometer, "that looks like a detonator."

He took out a small piece of paper, rubbed it over the inside and outside of the bag, then slid the paper into a special machine used to detect explosive residue. I passed.

"OK, you can go," he instructed. From then on, I would add a few extra minutes to my arrival time at the airport for my extra TSA inspection.

When they would call me out for a special bag check, I would kid with the inspector. "If you don't pull it out, you're not doing your job. I know because it looks like a bomb."

Some of the agents laughed, some didn't.

I was returning from one trip and my ice pack had melted, so the gel was soft and squishy. The TSA inspector pulled it out.

"I am going to have to confiscate this," she said. "It exceeds the three oz limit for liquids."

"But it's sealed and it's labeled *medical ice pack*," I protested. There is no reasoning with TSA agents—they are in charge. I relinquished the pack. From then on, I simply discarded the ice pack once I reached my destination. My secretary would call ahead to be sure that there was a refrigerator in my hotel room to keep my syringes cold. New ice packs arrived each month when the pharmacy supply company issued me a new quantity of medication. I would take these home to my freezer for later use. Two weeks after starting my injections, my CRP normalized and I began to feel normal most evenings.

"Living through better chemistry," I would tell my wife.

One of the major tenets of the *Affordable Care Act* (*ACA; Obamacare*) prohibited private insurance companies from excluding patients with pre-existing medical conditions from obtaining coverage. Having developed a chronic autoimmune condition, I wondered what people did before this legislation was passed? Did this prevent them from changing jobs secondary to fear of not being able to obtain health insurance coverage in their new position? Our most recent White House administration attempted unsuccessfully to repeal Obamacare with no real alternative being offered. This was narrowly defeated in the senate by one vote (may Senator John McCain rest in piece for being so bold!).

Three years went by and I had settled into a routine of daily injections and occasional TSA hassles. Then I had an exacerbation— the fever and malaise returned with a vengeance. We tried a short course of steroids like those often prescribed to treat poison ivy. No effect. We moved back to the original dose of high-dose oral steroids. A check of my *CRP* revealed a level of twenty-two (an all-time record for me)! I continued the daily injections and in combination with the steroids things settled down over the next two weeks. My repeat *CRP* was still elevated at four—not where I wanted it.

Reeves and I met to develop a plan. We agreed that the *anikara* was probably no longer working and it was time to switch to a new *monoclonal antibody* that had a different mechanism of action against *IL-1*. Because manufactured monoclonal antibodies are foreign to our bodies, we can actually form *neutralizing antibodies* to them. Go figure! The very immune system we are suppressing wakes up to block the therapy. Although there is no test for these antibodies, one can assume they are present when the medication stops working. I would need to start *canakinumab*, a different human *monoclonal antibody* that was first approved by the *FDA* for another rare autoimmune disease nine years earlier—*cryopyrin-associated periodic syndrome*.

There would be a big advantage. The medication would only be given once every one to two months. No more TSA hassle! A recent study had even shown a 15% reduction in the incidence of coronary heart disease in patients taking the drug. There was only one major drawback. The medication would cost $14,500 a month! We would have to get insurance approval for *off-label* use. Ten days later, I received a text from a pharmacy that handles injectable medications for my health insurance plan. They had not received approval for issuing the medication. My physician's office had not returned their inquiry as to the rationale for selecting this medication.

I undertook a series of eight phone calls that morning, with the final outcome being the pharmacy sending a request for a packet of information to my physician's office. One of the items was the need for a letter of medical necessity. The office nurse informed me that my physician was at a national meeting and that he would be difficult to reach. I offered to author the letter (I have written many of these in my time for my own patients) and send it to him by email for approval. Later that day, the pre-certification packet was returned to the pharmacy for consideration by the insurance company. They informed me that they would consider a seventy-two-hour urgent review; however, if I agreed to this, I would forfeit my right to a more prolonged review at a later date. We decided to go ahead with the rapid review.

Medications are approved by the FDA for specific diseases after extensive testing for safety in animals and later in human clinical trials. Once they are shown to be effective for a particular disease, they are released by the FDA for a specific indication. Physicians are allowed to use their clinical judgement to use this medication for other diseases if it proves effective. Such use is known as *off-label*. As an example, the FDA has only approved one drug for use in pregnancy—a progesterone injection to prevent premature delivery. All other medications used by OB-GYN's for various pregnancy conditions are used *off-label*.

Two weeks after my physician had ordered my new medication, it was shipped and appeared in a refrigerated portable cooler at my office. A new journey to live through better chemistry had begun.

20

A Significant Miss

Karen has been an obstetrical nurse for most of her adult life. After she finished nursing school, she worked on a Labor and Delivery Unit at a private hospital on the East Coast and then moved to the Labor and Delivery unit at the institution where I did my OB-GYN residency. After we were married in my last year of my OB-GYN residency, she took time off from nursing to raise my three daughters. Her fear of needles led to natural childbirth in all but the later stage of her first delivery. When she re-entered the nursing work force, she was instrumental in helping me establish fetal centers at four different institutions.

Karen had never been sick. The only time she was in a hospital was to deliver our three daughters. About four years ago, she began to experience severe pain and acid reflux with meals. We saw a gastroenterologist first. He recommended an upper GI endoscopy to look things over. In this procedure, they pass a lighted tube (*endoscope*) down your mouth to look at your *esophagus* (swallowing tube) and stomach. The good news is that they provide *conscious sedation* anesthesia (medication is given through an IV but a breathing tube is not used like they do for general anesthesia).

Karen was groggy in the recovery room from the anesthetic. The physician showed me the pictures he had taken through the scope.

"I got lost in the stomach," he told me. "Then I realized I was dealing with a large hernia."

After asking around, I found a premier *gastrointestinal (GI)* surgeon who specialized in *minimally invasive* surgery. Today, most surgeries are performed with small telescopes called *laparoscopes* through tiny incisions. The scope is connected to a camera that displays an image on multiple TV screens in the operating room. In most surgeries one to three instruments are placed through *ports* (plastic tubes) inserted through additional small abdominal incisions. These allow the surgeon to move, cut and *coagulate* (burn) tissues. In the case of abdominal surgery, carbon dioxide gas is used to inflate the abdomen to allow more room for the surgeon to operate. *Minimally invasive* surgery allows the patient to have the procedure performed as an *outpatient*. Because there is markedly less discomfort with the small incisions, the patient can be sent home the same day to recover once they are alert from their anesthesia.

In preparation for surgery, Karen had to undergo a CT scan and *esophageal manometry*. The CT scan was a breeze. It showed a large defect in the right side of the diaphragm with herniation of the stomach into the chest. The *manometry* was much worse. In this test, they put some numbing medicine in your nose and then spray the back of your throat with a numbing solution. They then pass a tube through your nose into your stomach. You are asked to swallow several gulps of water and the machine records the pressure waves as the fluid moves down from the mouth to the stomach. Karen has a deviated nasal septum. Passing the tube was not easy; it took five attempts. She told me later it was more painful than having a baby!

The surgeon decided Karen needed a *Nissan fundoplication.* He would pull the stomach out of the chest, fix the defect in the diaphragm, then wrap the esophagus around the entrance to the stomach to prevent acid reflux.

We were in the pre-operative area the day of surgery. Dr. Donner came by to make pre-op rounds.

"Any last-minute questions?" he asked.

"Say we never heard the results of the manometric study," I replied.

"Let's see," he said flipping through the chart. He paused for a moment. "This is a problem. I don't think we can do the *Nissen.* Your esophagus has been in your chest so long that it does not work properly. I am scared that if we do the *Nissen,* you may not be able to get solid food to pass the opening to the stomach."

Karen looked at me perplexed.

"And so what do we do?" I asked.

"Hmm, we can try the *Nissen,*" he replied. "If there is a problem we can always go back and do the more definitive operation."

"And what would that be?" I inquired.

"Well, we are talking about a much bigger operation to reroute your intestines," he replied.

My wife is one of the most strong-willed women I have met. She looked up at me as if to say, "Take me home."

Instead, she looked at me and said, "What should I do?"

"Well, this is your body. You have to decide," I replied.

"I can't. Decide for me," she instructed me.

"I know how much pain you have been in. I would go with the bigger surgery," I answered.

A new surgical consent had to be signed. Five hours later, Karen emerged from the operating room. All had gone well. We would spend the next twenty-four hours in the hospital dealing with her shoulder pain. It is not usual for patients that have undergone laparoscopic surgery to have pain between their neck and their shoulder. This is called *referred pain* and is related to the stretching of the lining of the abdomen from the carbon dioxide gas that was used at the surgery (even though most of it is taken out at the end of the case).

But on postoperative day two, the pain persisted.

"Probably related to those big stiches I put in to close the hole in the diaphragm," Donner said.

We went home that day and Karen made a slow recovery. She experienced bouts of nausea followed by diarrhea, so-called *dumping syndrome*. This is the residual effect of the intestinal surgery when sugars and fats pass rapidly through the small stomach straight into the intestines. With modifications to her diet, the symptoms eventually improved.

A year later, there was a recurrence of pain in Karen's upper abdomen. A repeat CT scan showed that the repair site was intact and the stomach was in the right position. But now the gallbladder was full of stones. Donner's associate performed an uneventful *laparoscopic cholecystectomy* (gall bladder removal). This time the surgery was performed as an outpatient and recovery was rapid.

Being a medical professional, Karen has always practiced preventative health care—Pap smears, mammograms, colonoscopy. Given a family history of heart disease, she decided to see a cardiologist to get a risk assessment. This included blood tests and a CT scan of the heart to look for calcifications—a marker for problems in the *coronary arteries* (the small arteries that supply blood to the heart). Her score came back in the low risk range. What the cardiologist did not inform her was that the CT scan had revealed a recurrence of the diaphragm hernia.

Six months later, Karen began to experience a repeat of her original symptoms. She returned to see Dr. Donner who ordered another CT scan. This showed a recurrence of the hernia with the small stomach pouch back in the chest. Are your symptoms bad enough to wait or do you want to move forward with a second repair?" he asked her. She elected to wait three months—then the symptoms worsened.

The second repair was more difficult than the first. The laparoscopic surgery took four hours. Dr. Donner repaired the right-sided defect in the diaphragm, made a relaxing incision in the left portion of the diaphragm to relieve any tension on the repair site, sutured a patch in place over the relaxing incision and then sutured the main portion of the stomach to the side of the abdomen to keep it in place. The most painful part was the big drain that remained in place for three days before it was removed.

Karen's recovery was slow. To complicate matters, Karen had to have a tooth pulled and a bone graft put in the socket for eventual placement of an implant. We called Donner to be sure it was OK to proceed with the bone graft. The mouth cavity is filled with bacteria and I was concerned that some of these could gain access to the bloodstream and implant on the diaphragm patch. This could result in a significant infection that would be difficult to treat. Donner gave us the green light on the bone graft.

It was now six weeks since the second diaphragm repair and Karen was still not bouncing back. She began to run a low-grade fever and complained about low back pain. A chiropractor treated her with massage and a roller machine; these made the pain worse. Her primary care physician thought the symptoms were related to stress and prescribed steroids.

On one occasion, she asked me to feel her lower back. "It feels like the fever is right here," she said.

I palpated her back and agreed that it felt warm. She went to visit our new granddaughter in North Carolina and I asked her get some blood tests at a local urgent care facility. They were sent to Donner—no problems that he could see.

"And she is too far out for this to be related to the surgery that I did," was his response.

I didn't accept this. As I mentioned earlier in the book, sometimes things have to progress to a point to where one finally releases control to an advocate—so-called *childhood regression*. Karen had finally reached that point.

A week later I decided to take her to see Donner.

"She is not getting better," I told him at the appointment.

"Well given the location of the pain I can only think of a *psoas abscess* (a collection of pus over one of the deep internal muscles of the back) which would be an unusual complication of the surgery. Let's get a CT," he suggested.

After the test, Karen returned to my apartment.

She called me at my office, "They want to admit me. They think they see an abscess on the CT."

We were in the hospital an hour later. Donner had called in an infectious disease expert—an older gentleman who was definitely old school. He sat at Karen's bedside and asked a wide array of questions.

"We will need to start you on some antibiotics and get a drain in this but it should be easily treatable," he reassured us.

"Here's the deal," I told Karen. "Since there was nothing on your pre-op CT just four months ago, this is got to be an abscess."

Dr. Donner appeared two hours later. He asked me to step out in the hall.

"I'm not sure this is an abscess," he said. "There are three radiologists looking at the films and they are still trying to figure this out."

Now I have looked at many CT scans and MRIs in my career. An abscess is usually easy to diagnose. Calling in three radiologists means something bad is there. My heart sank—it had to be some form of cancer.

"We will need to biopsy it. We will set it up for tomorrow," Donnor said.

"Let me talk to her," I asked.

I walked back into the hospital room trying to hold back tears.

"How honest do you want me to be with you?" I asked her.

"You need to tell me what's going on," she responded.

"It's not an abscess, it probably a tumor of some kind," I responded. "They will biopsy it tomorrow."

I hugged my wife of thirty-four years.

Through tears she implored me, "Promise me you will take care of our daughters and my mother".

"I promise", I replied.

I slept on the couch in the hospital room that night. Karen woke me up the next morning. "Am I reading this right?" she asked. "Come take a look. I accessed my patient portal to see the CT report from yesterday. It's not there but here is the report from the pre-op CT done two months ago."

I looked at the impression statement on the report: *1) A large diaphragm hernia is seen with stomach remnant in the chest 2) there is a suspicious periaortic lymph node seen. Clinical correlation is suggested.*

This statement is radiology lingo for "we don't like what we see and we suggest you look into it and do something about it". But nothing had been done. We had not even been told that this existed. This was clearly a *big miss.*

One of the unfortunate consequences of *HIPPA* legislation is that healthcare providers are now limited as to how they can communicate with their patients. In the past, I sent postcards to patients with the normal results of their annual pap smears. If there was a problem, the patient received a phone call. Today, texting and email correspondence with patients is taboo unless the messages use encryption software. Instead, the patients are instructed to use the *patient portal* as part of the EMR at that particular institution. This means that patients must maintain a password for each patient portal where they are seen. Laboratory and imaging results are automatically posted on the *portal* for the patient to check themselves. The responsibility for checking these results now falls to the patient. The old adage of "well the doctor's office did not call after the test, so everything must be fine" is no longer the case.

The biopsy was performed the next day using CT guidance to make sure the needle was in the right place. Despite sedation, Karen could hardly lay on her stomach due to her pain. We were sent home to await the results of the biopsy before we could determine the next step. The results came out forty-eight hours later – *large B cell, non-Hodgkin's lymphoma.*

Donner never apologized for his miss. In fact, I think the reason he first talked with me about the tumor was not that I was a physician, but that he had trouble facing Karen. Physicians are not taught to apologize for their mistakes. Karen was so angry she wanted to file a lawsuit. I talked with our oncologist later and he told me that the treatment she ultimately received would still have been the same based on the lymphoma cell type. This is true even though the tumor was much smaller on the pre-operative CT scan four months earlier.

I have three amazing daughters. They are genetically related to my wife and me but they could not have more different personalities. Rachael is the oldest. She lives on the East Coast with her husband and a daughter and a son. During the early phases of Karen's diagnosis, I was in constant contact with her by phone to keep her up-to-date. I was able to sit down with my third daughter, Erin, the following weekend to tell her about Karen's diagnosis. Until then, she was under the impression that this was some form of infection.

"It's not," I told her. "Mom has a form of cancer. It is a lymphoma."

She looked at me bewildered then burst into tears. After almost six years of trying different vocations after college graduation, Erin had applied to PA school and just been accepted after the first round of interviews. She had an immediate reaction to the news about her mother.

Through sobbing tears she told me, "I'm not going to school. I am going to stay home to take care of Mom."

"That's not what she would want for you. I have Mom's back. We want you to start PA school," I responded.

Breaking the news to my second-born daughter, Kaitlyn, would be the most difficult. She is the most emotional of my three daughters. She lives in Manhattan where she has been pursuing her dream of dancing and acting. We would have to do this by phone. Karen called her fiancée, Nathan, and asked him to be at her apartment when we placed the call. It would have to be a few days later to match up with their schedules.

At the scheduled time, I dialed the number but Karen would not take the phone.

"I can't do this; you have to talk to her," Karen said.

"Kaitlyn, how are you?" I said.

"Doing fine Dad, what's up?" she replied.

"Well I have something to talk to you about, "I said holding back tears. "You know Mom had that biopsy the other day."

The phone went silent.

"We just got the results back and it is a lymphoma," I said.

"What does that mean?" she asked.

"Well, it's a form of cancer," I answered.

The crying over the phone tore my heart from my chest.

"Is Mom going to die?" she asked.

"The doctor says that the chemotherapy treatment has a good chance for a response," I said. "Well I am not getting married," she replied.

"No, that's not what we want for you," I said.

"I need to speak to Mom," she implored me through tears.

She and Karen talked for a while. Karen reassured her that she would be fine and that she planned on being around to celebrate grandchildren. I talked with Nathan later at their wedding eight months later. He told me Kaitlyn had cried inconsolably for the next four hours before she finally fell asleep. I told him how much we appreciated him being there for her.

I have never been a fan of tattoos. As an OB-GYN, I have often discovered tattoos in the most unusual of places. For the most part, my patients were always sorry they had these. Many remember getting them with their classmates on a college spring break. When my girls were young, I had shared my aversion to tattoos with them.

"Dad has a belt sander in the garage he can use to remove the tattoo if I find it," I warned them. That seemed to do the trick.

But we decided in an act of solidarity that we would all get a tattoo once Karen had completed her therapy. I suggested we use the cancer institute's logo—the word "cancer" with a line drawn through it. This would be good advertisement for the hospital with the whole family showing off their tattoos. Karen didn't like the idea.

"How about the Zodiac cancer sign with an arrow through it?" I queried.

Turns out the Zodiac sign for cancer is a crab. My girls refused to have a crab tattooed on their bodies. My third daughter had a brilliant suggestion—the cancer star constellation is three outer stars surrounding by a central star. Perfect—each outer star would represent one of our daughters with their mom in the center. We could put an arrow through the constellation signaling we had defeated cancer. Rachael would get a designer to draw the picture. I would have to be first in line for the tattoo. I agreed.

It came time to share Karen's diagnosis with my Chairman and colleagues. After all, it would have an impact on my work schedule. Many knew Karen from her previous association with our Fetal Center. The most common response I received was "I am so sorry." While the intent of this response is clearly meant to be caring, I began to hear it so often that it began to rapidly lose its meaning. I would much rather that friends and colleagues ask what they could do for us.

We were lucky. There is a world-renowned cancer institute in our town. I picked up the phone even before the final biopsy results had returned to schedule an appointment in the lymphoma clinic—it would be a three-week wait. Meanwhile Karen's discomfort continued to worsen. So, I called a pediatric *hematologist* (a specialist in blood disorders) I knew and asked if he had any colleagues at the cancer institute where he could call in a favor. Karen got a phone call about a work-in appointment the following week. In the interim, I contacted the first hospital where we had the biopsy and asked for a set of the slides from the biopsy to be sent to the cancer institute.

My oldest daughter had started a blog on CaringBridge—an amazing website for patients and support persons to get the updates to family and friends. This was an angel wink for me. I entered updates into the blog almost every day to let friends and family know our progress. They all sent amazing messages and prayers to Karen which I would share with her.

When we finally met our *hemoncologist* (a specialist who takes care of patients with cancers related to blood cells), the slides had not arrived for review by the institute's pathologist.

"Not unusual," Dr. Ayed said. "They look upon us as their competition. They usually drag their feet on sending over the slides."

"Really?" I asked. "And in a patient with cancer?"

Dr. Ayed was not one of those touchy-feely physicians. He was somewhat reassuring however.

"I used to take care of patients with solid tumors," he said. "I got frustrated because I could not cure my patients. I moved to liquid tumors (*lymphomas, leukemias, multiple myeloma*) because I can cure these."

This seemed like a ray of hope. He told use that Karen had some good things going for her—she was healthy and less than sixty years of age. The prognosis for non-Hodgkin's lymphoma is better for patients under sixty years of age.

"By only three months," Karen pointed out.

"Yes, but we will take that," he replied.

The first step in the evaluation would be a bone marrow biopsy.

"Just a small bump," he assured Karen. I knew better. This would be followed by a *PET scan*. A *PET scan* is used in some cancer cases to detect actively dividing cells. A radioactive substance is injected into the patient's vein and then a special CT scan is done to detect the "hot spots" that indicate the location of the cancer cells.

We started with the bone marrow biopsy. It was done in a special clinic as an outpatient. In a bone marrow biopsy, the patient's skin over the back of the pelvic bone is injected with a numbing medication. A needle that is twice as big as the one use to draw blood from a patient's arm is then inserted into the bone and blood is drawn into a syringe. After this, the bone marrow biopsy is done. A new needle is inserted (three and a half times larger than the needle used to draw blood) back into the bone to core out a cylinder of bone.

What was interesting was that a *physician associate (PA)* not an MD performed the procedure. Future efforts to curb the cost of health care will include the use of a growing number of allied health professionals in the direct care of patients. The education of physicians is costly and requires eleven to thirteen years depending on subspecialty specialization. Allied health professionals work under the direct supervision of physicians and cannot practice independently:

Physician associate (PA): four years college, two years PA school—inpatient and outpatient clinical work

Nurse practitioner (NP): four years college, two years nursing experience, two to four years NP school (master's degree)—most outpatient clinical work

Nurse anesthetist (CRNA): four years college, one to two years ICU or ER nursing experience, two to three years CRNA school (masters or doctorate degree)—inpatient and outpatient surgeries.

This PA at the cancer institute probably did thirty bone marrows every day. After all, that was the only thing she did. On the particular day that Karen was scheduled, the lead PA was training another PA to do the procedure. Karen has been in healthcare most of her adult life but is deathly afraid of needles.

"I need to pull the medicine card," she stated. "I don't want a learner."

The senior PA did the procedure.

About thirty minutes later, Karen returned to the waiting room with an angry look on her face.

"What's wrong?" I asked.

"They told me that I can have *conscious sedation* next time if I have to have this done again," she replied.

The next step was the *PET scan*. Easy enough. Then back to the lymphoma clinic a week later.

Dr. Ayed walked in with bad news. The tissue slides from the first hospital were of too poor quality to perform all the necessary analysis. We would have to repeat the biopsy. Worse news—the bone marrow biopsy did not contain enough tissue. It would have to be repeated as well. We would also need an MRI to evaluate Karen's spine since the *PET scan* showed possible spinal canal involvement.

The next week we were back to the cancer hospital. Both the repeat bone marrow and the repeat *CT-directed lymph node biopsy* were done under *conscious sedation* (patients receive intravenous medications under the care of an anesthesiologist that comes close to putting them asleep).

I called the oncologist's office and asked if we could go ahead and place the special port catheter that would be used for chemotherapy. Chemotherapy is typically given as a medication in a vein. If these toxic medications leak outside of the vein, they can cause a large burn with loss of tissue. For this reason, patients getting intense chemotherapy often have a special plastic tube placed in the large vein under their collar bone. The tube is tunneled under the skin to a *port*—a cylinder that is placed under the skin. To give the chemotherapy, a needle is placed through the skin into the *port*. The surgeon at the cancer institute who placed the port was comical. He told us he had placed over 10,000 ports. Reassuring—he would probably have that infamous muscle memory and have few complications.

"I will talk with you during the case to tell you what I am doing," he told Karen.

"I prefer you wait to talk with me until after I am in the recovery room," she replied. If you can do this surgery without pain, I'll talk with you about marriage," she replied.

The port placement went well. A few days later, the MRI turned out to be the easiest procedure of the week.

We returned to see Dr. Ayed the next week. The whole process seemed to be taking forever. Karen's pain was well controlled with minimal narcotics but she still ran fevers every night and had no appetite. The biopsy showed a *large-cell GCB lymphoma* with *double expression* for two cell markers. This signified a more aggressive type of lymphoma with a poorer prognosis. Instead of the usual outpatient chemotherapy (called *R-CHOP* for the abbreviation of the chemother-apy agents in this regimen), we would need to have inpatient drugs for six cycles every three weeks. This regimen was dubbed *R-EPOCH*. Each cycle would last five days and Karen would get four drugs and one monoclonal antibody as part of *immunotherapy*. And the worse news—each cycle would include a spinal tap with a fifth drug injected to be sure that no cancer cells were in the spinal fluid.

In the meantime, I was pouring over as much information as I could find on non-Hodgkin's lymphoma. The pregnant patients I care for are young and my only experience with cancer in this popu-lation was an occasional breast cancer patient. I knew little about lymphoma. I was concerned about the nausea and vomiting with the chemotherapy. Karen still had some residual issues with nausea after certain meals due to the revision of her intestines that she had previously undergone. The *National Comprehensive Cancer Network* (NCC) had published guidelines on what medications should be used to prevent nausea and vomiting based on the *emetic* (nausea-in-ducing) potential of the chemotherapy[94]. Karen was scheduled to get two of the drugs that were ranked as having high emetic poten-tial—more than a 90% chance for severe nausea. I presented these guidelines to Dr. Ayed and asked if Karen could receive one of the newer anti-emetic medications—*aprepitant (Emend®)*, a neurokinin-1 receptor blocker.

Well, we usually start with *ondansetron (Zofran®)* and see how she does with the first cycle," he said. "If she does not do well, we can use that medication on the next cycle."

It is a well-known phenomenon that once a chemotherapy patient experiences extreme nausea, they will have *anticipatory emesis* when it is time for the next round of chemotherapy. This is very difficult to prevent. The brain simply knows what is to come—a form of post-traumatic stress disorder.

I pushed back. "Well you know Karen has ongoing issues with nausea with her previous surgery," I said. "I really don't want to see her get behind with just *ondansetron*. And besides, the NCC guideline states that the chemotherapy that Karen will receive will be in the high-risk emetic category and that *aprepitant* is indicated," I said.

Ayed responded, "At our cancer institute we don't always follow the national guidelines on all occasions."

"Yes, but one of your faculty was on the committee that wrote these guidelines," I answered. Ayed relented. Karen received *aprepitant* at the start of each of her six cycles. She had no nausea throughout her chemotherapy. The episode taught me that I would have to be her advocate for the next few months.

We were admitted for our first treatment that same day. We waited twelve hours to get into a bed. The *rituximab* (*Rituxan®*) was first. *Rituximb* is a man-made *monoclonal antibody* that attaches to lymphoma cells and causes one's own immune system to attach and kill the cells. We could expect a pretty severe reaction with the first dose due to the size of Karen's lymphoma mass. The only problem is that it also causes what is known as an *acute inflammatory state*—the release of chemicals into the blood stream that causes fever, chills, and changes in blood pressure.

The nurse started the medication at 11 p.m. A half hour later, Karen had a fever to 103 and the hospital bed was shaking with her chills. Her reaction to this treatment will probably be one of those memories that I will take to my grave. As an obstetrician, it was not easy to watch my wife deal with the pain of labor through three bouts of natural childbirth with our three daughters. This was so much worse. It was terrible to watch and I felt so helpless. They gave Karen a dose of intravenous narcotic to stop the chills and then slowed the infusion.

The nurse turned to me, "This is a good thing. It means the cancer cells are dying. It won't be as bad next time around."

Karen barely remembered the events of the first night in the hospital. The next day. I explained what had happened.

"I don't remember any of that," she said. "But I remember the three visitors at the foot of my bed."

"But there was only the nurse and me in the room last night," I responded.

"No, there were three strangers standing at the foot of my bed," she said. "One was a man and two were women. They were dressed in white and did not speak. They simply stood there and watched over me. I felt a sense of calm that they were sent to take care of me."

The hair on the back of my neck stood up. This would be the first of many signs to come that a greater power was sending messengers to guide Karen through her treatment.

The next day, the first round of chemotherapy was started. Karen joked that the *etoposide (Veposid®)* was her champagne (it had lots of bubbles) and the *doxorubicin (Adriamycin®)* was her rosé wine (it was a red mixture). The steroids they added as part of the treatment had Karen all jazzed up. She had problems sleeping but the meds we had selected to prevent nausea were working well so her appetite was good.

And then it was time for the first spinal tap. Since the lymphoma had eroded into the front side of one of her vertebrae, chemotherapy would be injected into the spinal canal to kill any cancer cells that may have migrated there. Karen has an overwhelming fear of needles. I think the fear of an epidural needle in her back is probably the reason she chose natural childbirth with our three daughters.

A PA did the spinal tap and did a fantastic job of talking Karen through the whole procedure. She even admitted that she was just as fearful of needles.

Throughout the rounds of chemotherapy, I worked in my clinic most days since my hospital was only a few blocks away. Each afternoon I would return to sleep in Karen's room. I learned to hate the *etoposide* infusion. It was mixed in a solution that caused microbubbles to form. These would get caught in the infusion pump and make it alarm due to an occlusion. Since the nurses could not hear the alarm at the nursing station, we would have to call for the nurse on the bedside control to have her come to the room to fix the infusion pump. This would occur six to seven times nightly—a pain for the nurses and even more of a problem for the cancer patient trying to get some sleep. I didn't get much sleep either.

On the third night of our first round of chemotherapy, I heard Karen begin to cough. I have always taught OB-GYN residents that a new onset of cough in an otherwise healthy patient is an early sign of *pulmonary edema* (extra fluid accumulating in the air spaces of the lungs).

I went to the night nurse. She probably thought I was a bit crazy but she knew I was a physician.

"Can we look at Karen's *I & O's* (the amount of fluid given to the patient and the amount she has urinated)?" I asked.

She calculated these with me. Karen was four liters ahead (almost a gallon of extra fluid).

"Can you come listen to her lungs?" I asked.

She heard *rales*—a crackling sound heard in the lungs with a stethoscope indicating *pulmonary edema*.

"Can you call the oncology fellow and see if we can get her some Lasix® to make her pee some of this off?" I asked.

After the medication, Karen put out three liters of urine. I will always wonder what would have happened if I was an average lay support person. Would Karen have ended up in the intensive care unit?

The rest of the first cycle went well. Since all the infusions were timed, Karen had figured out the exact time they would all be completed. Our bags were packed and we were ready to go home even before the attending physician had a chance to come by to make rounds that final morning.

Probably the best medicine that Karen received were the visits from her old friends. Many belonged to a select group of moms that had bonded during the years when their children and ours were all in the same elementary school. Old friendships were re-kindled. One of Karen's old friends stopped by and brought her a nursing bra—a welcome solution to the problem of needing access to the IV port in the upper part of her chest.

By the time of the third hospital admission for chemotherapy, I had grown tired of sleepless nights from *etoposide* microbubbles. Karen would not let me open the infusion pump to tap the line to remove the bubbles like the nurses were doing, so the nursing calls through the night continued. One evening, we took a trip to the top floor of the hospital where there was an indoor observation deck. Several of the patients receiving inpatient chemotherapy were there visiting with friends and family. One teenager was playing cards with several friends. She was getting the same chemotherapy as Karen—I recognized the color of her medication bags that were hanging on the

IV pole. Sure enough, a few minutes later her infusion pump began to alarm from the microbubbles in the *etoposide*. She turned it off, took the IV tubing out of the infusion pump, tapped it a few times to get the bubbles to move up, and then started the pump back.

"See," I pointed out to Karen. "Even a teenager can do this."

We returned to the room and while Karen was napping I decided to Google "*etoposide* and microbubbles." Much to my surprise an oncology nursing website popped up. It described how the nurses at another major cancer institute in New York had solved the problem with a simple anti-siphon filter. I Googled the company that made the filter. Back at my office the next day, I printed both websites.

Later that next afternoon, I asked if I could meet with the charge nurse on the floor. When she arrived, I told her what I had found.

"Well, we tried one of those filters a while back and it didn't solve the problem," she said. "I will take the information and bring it to our practice committee. But change is slow around here."

After the third cycle of chemotherapy, Karen underwent a repeat PET scan—great news, the tumors were markedly decreased in volume. The cancer was responding!

We were headed back to our home a few hours away from the cancer institute. On the way, we stopped by a roadside bakery that has been a fixture of the community for over one hundred years. We were sitting down to a sandwich when a woman walked up to Karen. Karen's friend had shaved her head to keep the rest of her hair from falling out from the chemotherapy. She was wearing a bandana.

"I know you are undergoing chemotherapy," the stranger said. "I had breast cancer last year and I lost my hair too. It will grow back even better than before when you finish your treatment. Can I pray over you?" she asked.

She placed her hands on Karen's head and prayed for her recovery. Then she walked away. We both looked at one other—another angel had been sent into our lives to send us a message; everything was going to be OK.

By the fourth chemotherapy cycle, we were real veterans of the process. Karen would check in with bed control soon after we arrived for our oncology appointment. We would be seen by Dr. Ayed and then admitted a few hours later. I would go back to the car and get our supplies. We had learned a lot about what we needed in the hospital room. I arrived with a small canvas wagon filled with multiple tiers of belongings—a coffee pot, an aroma aerosol machine, pillows, an egg crate mattress for my bed couch—all the comforts of home.

By the fourth cycle, I had befriended the little lady who took the payment for the overnight valet parking at the hospital.

She would ask me each morning when I would check in to get my car to drive to my clinic, "Do you have surgery today, Doc?"

If I responded yes, she would call over to the parking attendants, "Heh, Doc needs his car right away for surgery. Let's get that here ASAP."

The *etoposide* bubbles in the hospital continued to haunt us. It had been three weeks and no news from the charge nurse who promised to get back to me. I needed to take it up a notch. I wrote a letter to the president of the cancer institute on my university letterhead. This was not only a problem for the nursing staff, it was a problem for the patients. I concluded my letter by pointing out that it was nursing week—what a way to honor those who worked so hard to care for the oncology patients if we could solve the constant need to fix the infusion pumps. The next day the chief nursing officer of the hospital came to our room. I told her the story of the teenager on the observation deck that had taken care of the bubbles in her own infusion pump. She was not pleased—a real liability for the hospital. I gave her copies of the information I had discovered on the internet. She promised me that by Karen's next cycle, the institution would order a few of the filters and we would be the pilot study.

Cycle five arrived. The wagon was piled even higher this time with personal effects for our admission. I had to make two trips to the car. When the infusion nurse came in, she proudly showed us the new filter for the *etoposide*. That night, the infusion pump did not alarm even once! No alarms the next day as well. We became instant celebrities on the floor. This problem had plagued the institution for years and we had solved it with a simple internet search. I wrote a follow-up letter to thank the president of the institution for his rapid response to my inquiry. Last I heard, the Director of nursing told me that they were planning to implement the filter on all of their hospital floors. As someone once said, "The squeakee wheel gets the oil."

Medicine has become a competitive business. Hospitals compete for the infamous "best in class" ratings in various specialties that are published annually by *U.S. News and World Report*[95]. Billboards are strategically placed on highways that commuters use to enter the city every day to advertise these rankings. Websites and television commercials tout the rankings as well. A study recently found that hospitals nationwide spend more than $5.6 million annually on advertising[96]. This competition of course has its downside. Hospitals are not willing to share their best practices to improve patient care. The *etoposide* filter had clearly been an example of this.

Cycle six finally arrived. At the end of a chemotherapy regimen, it is customary at most cancer hospitals to "ring the bell." This is to signal that life has started again. Karen and I had heard several of the bell ringings while we were in the hospital but this one would be special for us. All of the floor nurses routinely showed up and clap

Kenneth J. Moise, Jr. M.D.

for the patient. Unfortunately, we did not finish our last infusion until almost 10 p.m.. Nevertheless, it was an emotional moment. We face-timed our girls and my middle daughter was in tears as she watched her mom ring the bell to signal her new lease on life. Then we packed up for the last time and headed out.

I stopped by the valet parking area and give my favorite cashier a gift card for Starbucks.

"I hate to say this but I hope not to see you any time soon," I said to her.

She smiled at me and replied, "I understand."

Our third daughter would have her *white coat ceremony* the following Friday—she would get her first white coat and take her professional oath as a physician associate. Classes would start soon thereafter.

The following week we returned for our repeat PET scan—it was all clear—we were in remission. It was time to schedule the family tattoos.

356

21

Epilogue

Kathy's Rh disease would require at least four more intrauterine transfusions of her unborn baby girl after that Thanksgiving trip from Florida.

"After my last pregnancy when my OB basically abandoned me, I am not sure I can trust anyone in Florida to take care of me," she said. But on my fireman's salary, I don't know how I can afford to fly back and forth to see you for all the procedures."

Karen stepped in. "Let me work on it," she responded.

She contacted *Angel Flight*—a group of volunteer pilots that fly patients for medical care at no charge. It would take two flights between Florida and our medical center. Kathy would have to change planes in Atlanta because of the distance. We could plan to house her at the *Ronald McDonald House* near our medical center. Calling on her fireman fraternity of brothers, they came through to pick her up from our local airport each trip and transport her to and from the hospital. Four intrauterine transfusions later, her baby girl, Madison, had turned the corner and we were getting close to time for delivery.

"I want you to deliver Madison," Kathy pleaded.

"It would be an honor," I answered. "She should only have to stay in the hospital for a few days after she is born. Then we can get both of you back home to Florida for good."

Three weeks later Kathy returned to our hospital and I induced her labor. Things went well and she had an uncomplicated vaginal delivery. Three days later, mom and baby returned home together for the last time—this time Madison traveled in Kathy's arms. Every year at Christmas I receive a special card with a photo of Madison with a *Thank you, Dr. Moise* inscription.

Medicine has changed our lives. An individual born in the USA in 1990 lived on average to age forty-seven. One in seven babies born in 2020 will live to be over 100[97]. All of us will develop an illness at some point in our lives. Ultimately all of us will die. The science of medicine has advanced so rapidly. Only ninety years have passed since Alexander Fleming discovered the first antibiotic—penicillin. Today we are on the brink of correcting inherited genetic defects with *CRISPIR-Cas9* technology, a method of inserting a gene into a cell. This has already been employed in patients with sickle cell anemia and thalassemia for a cure[98]. Personalized medicine is the new buzz word in healthcare. Therapies are designed for individual patients based on the genetics of a cancer or the patient's overall genetic makeup. One such example is *CART-T* cell therapy. Immune cells are harvested from lymphoma patients and then genetically modified to be better attack agents. They are then reinfused back into the patient where they were first taken. Spina bifida in fetuses is now being surgically corrected in the womb through tiny telescopes called *fetoscopes*. In the near future, artificial intelligence in computers will probably replace the need for radiologists to read images or the need for pathologists to interpret tissue slides to make a diagnosis.

But with all these advances, comes a price. How do we afford the costs of continued progress? One of the basic tenets is to decide if healthcare is a *privilege* or a *right*. I would argue that it is the *right* of the individual. The next challenge is how to pay for this *right*. One can adopt a socialistic view that all should contribute to a universal healthcare system much like that in Sweden or Canada. Recent politicians have even proposed a "Medicare for all" concept. Several issues are lost in this argument. The first is that the population of countries with socialized health care is generally homogenous, much different than the broad diversity of the American populous. The second is that the population of Sweden is 3% the size of the U.S. population and the Canadian population is only 10% as large. Finally, and most importantly, is the concept of personal freedom—one of the founding premises of our country. Some individuals choose to purchase a jeep for transportation and some can afford a Maserati. For this reason, I do not believe that a government-run, single-payor system will ever be accepted by the American public.

A hospital CEO one day at lunch told me his vision of the U.S. healthcare system. "I think it's like a commercial airline flight," he said. "The pilots are seated in the front and fly the plane. There is a first-class part of the cabin. Passengers pay more for a seat and get special food and services. In the rear of the plane is coach. The seats are smaller and there are no meals, only a beverage. But the pilots fly the entire plane. Everyone arrives at their destination safely."

We physicians are the best advocates for our patients. We believe that basic healthcare is a *right* not a *privilege*. All patients should have access to basic healthcare, especially in catastrophic circumstances—an auto accident or a new diagnosis of cancer. I do not have all the answers, but I worry that politicians do not understand that the healthcare system must change slowly with significant input from the providers in the trenches. After all it occupies almost one-fifth of our gross domestic product. As I described earlier in the book, the governmental effort to incentivize the EMR has been an overall failure leading to increased costs and physician burnout.

As I look forward to my last few years in medicine, I can peer back on my contributions and hope I will be judged as having made a difference. I have tried to teach my students the art and the science of medicine. I have tried to provide the best care for my patients. And I hope I demonstrated some vision and have affected some small change in the science of medicine just a little. If I have accomplished all of this, I can retire with a glint in my eye for eventually I too one day will become the patient.

BIBLIOGRAPHY

Chapter 2

1. Hirshfield LE, Yudkowsky R, Park YS. Pre-medical majors in the humanities and social sciences: impact on communication skills and specialty choice. Med Educ. 2019;53(4):408-16.

2. Youngclaus JJ, Frresne AJ, Bunton, AS. An updated look at attendance cost and medical student debt at US medical schools. PDX Scholar, 2017.

3. $100 Million Gift Makes NYU Medical School Free [Available from: https://www.capturehighered.com/nyu-medical-school-free/].

Chapter 3

4. Macdonald GJ, MacGregor DB. Procedures for embalming cadavers for the dissecting laboratory. Proc Soc Exp Biol Med. 1997;215(4):363-5.

5. Zampieri F, ElMaghawry M, Zanatta A, Thiene G. Andreas Vesalius: Celebrating 500 years of dissecting nature. Glob Cardiol Sci Pract. 2015;2015(5):66.

Chapter 4

6. Murphy B. Why some medical students are cutting
    class to get ahead. { Available from: https://www.
    ama-assn.org/medical-students/medical-school-life/
    why-some-medical-students-are-cutting-class-get-ahead].

7. Dumont M. [The forceps. History. Current indications]. Rev
    Fr Gynecol Obstet. 1988;83(4):220-5.

Chapter 5

8. Wentz DK, Ford CV. A brief history of the internship. JAMA.
    1984;252(24):3390-4.

9. Accredication Council for Graduate Medical Education.
    Glossary of Terms. [Available from: http://acgme.org/
    acgmeweb/Portals/0/PFAssets/ProgramRequirements/ab_
    ACGMEglossary.pdfa].

10. Chervenak FA, Asfaw TS, Shaktman BD, McCullough
    LB. Gender diversity in residency training: The case for
    affirmative Iiclusion. J Grad Med Educ. 2017;9(6):685-7.

11. Association of American Medical Colleges. The majority of
    U.S. medical students are women, new data show [Available
    from: https://www.aamc.org/news-insights/press-
    releases/majority-us-medical-students-are-women-new-
    data-show#:~:text=The%20proportion%20of%20women%20
    students,of%20all%20medical%20school%20students.&tex-
    t=Across%20applicants%20and%20matriculants%2C%20
    the,the%20number%20of%20men%20declined.

12. Statista. Percentage of physicians in select specialties
    in the U.S. who were women as of 2020 [Available

from: https://www.statista.com/statistics/1019841/
female-physicians-women-specialties-us/].

13. Certification of laboratories 1988 [Available from: https://
www.govinfo.gov/content/pkg/USCODE-2011-title42/
pdf/USCODE-2011-title42-chap6A-subchapII-partF-
subpart2-sec263a.pdf].

14. Michaels PA. A chapter from lamaze history: birth narratives
and authoritative knowledge in france, 1952-1957. J Perinat
Educ. 2010;19(2):35-43.

15. Varner CA. Comparison of the Bradley method and
hypnoBirthing childbirth education classes. J Perinat Educ.
2015;24(2):128-36.

16. Silva M, Halpern SH. Epidural analgesia for labor: Current
techniques. Local Reg Anesth. 2010;3:143-53.

17. Xu J, Murphy SL, Kochanek KD, E. A. Births: Final Data for
2019. Nt Vit Statis Report. 2021;70:1-86.

Chapter 7

18. Lasagna LA. A modern Hippocratic Oath. Tuft Med All Bull.
1986;46:34.

19. Nixon, J. Ten years of tort reform in Texas: A review. The
Heritage Foundation, (Available from: http://report.
heritage.org/bg2830].

20. Paik M, Black BS, Hyman DA, Silver C. Will tort ferform
bend the cost curve? Evidence from Texas. JoEmp Legal Stud.
2012;9:1-44.

Kenneth J. Moise, Jr. M.D.

21. Guardado JR. New data show the highest prevalence of medical liability premium increases in 15 Years 2021 [Available from: https://www.ama-assn.org/system/files/2021-03/prp-mlm-premiums-2020.pdf].

Chapter 9

22. Liley AW. Intrauterine transfusion of foetus in haemolytic disease. Br Med J. 1963;2(5365):1107-9.

Chapter 10

23. American College of Obsetricians and Gynecologists, Society for Maternal-Fetal Medicine, Menard MK, Kilpatrick S, Saade G, et al. Levels of maternal care. Am J Obstet Gynecol. 2015;212(3):259-71.

24. Petrilli CM, Saint S, Jennings JJ, Caruso A, Kuhn L, Snyder A, et al. Understanding patient preference for physician attire: a cross-sectional observational study of 10 academic medical centres in the USA. BMJ Open. 2018;8(5):e021239.

Chapter 11

25. Muraskas J, Parsi K. The cost of saving the tiniest lives: NICUs versus prevention. Virtual Mentor. 2008;10(10):655-8.

26. Levin DL, Mills LJ, Parkey M, Garriott J, Campbell W. Constriction of the fetal ductus arteriosus after administration of indomethacin to the pregnant ewe. J Pediatr. 1979;94(4):647-50.

27. Huhta JC, Moise KJ, Fisher DJ, Sharif DS, Wasserstrum N, Martin C. Detection and quantitation of constriction of

the fetal ductus arteriosus by Doppler echocardiography. Circulation. 1987;75(2):406-12.

28. Moise KJ, Jr., Huhta JC, Sharif DS, Ou CN, Kirshon B, Wasserstrum N, et al. Indomethacin in the treatment of premature labor. Effects on the fetal ductus arteriosus. N Engl J Med. 1988;319(6):327-31.

29. Bang J, Bock JE, Trolle D. Ultrasound-guided fetal intravenous transfusion for severe rhesus haemolytic disease. Br Med J 1982;284(6313):373-4.

30. Daffos F, Capella-Pavlovsky M, Forestier F. Fetal blood sampling via the umbilical cord using a needle guided by ultrasound. Report of 66 cases. Prenat Diagn. 1983;3(4):271-7.

31. Parisi VM, Salinas J, Stockmar EJ. Fetal vascular responses to maternal nicardipine administration in the hypertensive ewe. Am J Obstet Gynecol. 1989;161(4):1035-9.

32. Moise KJ, Jr., Ou CN, Kirshon B, Cano LE, Rognerud C, Carpenter RJ, Jr. Placental transfer of indomethacin in the human pregnancy. Am J Obstet Gynecol. 1990;162(2):549-54.

33. Berger RL. Nazi science—the Dachau hypothermia experiments. N Engl J Med. 1990;322(20):1435-40.

34. Rusert B. "A study in nature": the Tuskegee experiments and the New South plantation. J Med Humanit. 2009;30(3):155-71.

35. Culliton BJ. National research act: restores training, bans fetal research. Science. 1974;185(4149):426-7.

36. Sims JM. A brief review of the Belmont report. Dimens Crit Care Nurs. 2010;29(4):173-4.

37. Nosowsky R, Giordano TJ. The Health Insurance Portability and Accountability Act of 1996 (HIPAA) privacy rule: implications for clinical research. Annu Rev Med. 2006;57:575-90.

38. Raffle AE, Gray JM. The 1960s cervical screening incident at National Women's Hospital, Auckland, New Zealand: insights for screening research, policy making, and practice. J Clin Epidemiol. 2020;122:A8-A13.

39. Wohn Y. Research misconduct. Seoul National University dismisses Hwang. Science. 2006;311(5768):1695.

Chapter 12

40. Medpage Today . Schwarzenegger's aortic valve replacement [Available from: https://www.medpagetoday.com/ popmedicine/celebritydiagnosis/89475].

41. Bill and Melinda Gates Foundation GoalKeepers. Maternal Mortality [Available from: https://www.gatesfoundation. org/goalkeepers/report/2021-report/progress-indicators/ maternal-mortality/].

42. World Health Organization . Maternal Deaths [Available from: https://www.who.int/data/gho/ indicator-metadata-registry/imr-details/4622].

Chapter 13

43. Merkatz IR, Nitowsky HM, Macri JN, Johnson WE. An association between low maternal serum alpha-fetoprotein and fetal chromosomal abnormalities. Am J Obstet Gynecol. 1984;148(7):886-94.

44. W.K. Kellogg Foundation. Doulas: Ancient practice helps solve a modern crisis [Available from: https://everychildthrives.com/doulas-ancient-practice-helps-solve-a-modern-crisis/?gclid=CjwKCAiAnZCdBhBmEiwA8nDQxYKz7EykmFkIPV2Ty1YdFazYuWbrIv89Wwj4QYm5T-F0tYBMiGADVhoCHI8QAvD_BwE].

45. Akolekar R, Beta J, Picciarelli G, Ogilvie C, D'Antonio F. Procedure-related risk of miscarriage following amniocentesis and chorionic villus sampling: a systematic review and meta-analysis. Ultrasound Obstet Gynecol. 2015;45(1):16-26.

46. Vintzileos AM, Egan JF, Smulian JC, Campbell WA, Guzman ER, Rodis JF. Adjusting the risk for trisomy 21 by a simple ultrasound method using fetal long-bone biometry. Obstet Gynecol. 1996;87(6):953-8.

47. Bahado-Singh RO, Tan A, Deren O, Hunter D, Copel J, Mahoney MJ. Risk of Down syndrome and any clinically significant chromosome defect in pregnancies with abnormal triple-screen and normal targeted ultrasonographic results. Am J Obstet Gynecol. 1996;175:824-9.

48. Nicolaides KH, Azar G, Byrne D, Mansur C, Marks K. Fetal nuchal translucency: ultrasound screening for chromosomal defects in first trimester of pregnancy. BMJ. 1992;304(6831):867-9.

49. Nicolaides KH, Syngelaki A, Ashoor G, Birdir C, Touzet G. Noninvasive prenatal testing for fetal trisomies in a routinely screened first-trimester population. Am J Obstet Gynecol. 2012;207(5):374 e1-6.

50. Cheng YW, Snowden JM, King TL, Caughey AB. Selected perinatal outcomes associated with planned home births in the United States. Am J Obstet Gynecol. 2013;209(4):325 e1-8.

Chapter 14

51. Time. Peacock's *Dr. Death* Is Based on a Chilling True Crime Podcast About a Murderous Surgeon. Here's What to Know [Available from: https://time.com/6080714/dr-death-true-story/].

52. Kohn LT, Corrigan JM. To Err is Human. Buliding a safer health system: Institute of Medicine; 2000.

53. Perell D. Why did the Boeing 737 Max crash? [Available from: https://perell.com/essay/boeing-737-max/].

54. Bendavid E, Kaganova Y, Needleman J, Gruenberg L, Weissman JS. Complication rates on weekends and weekdays in US hospitals. Am J Med. 2007;120(5):422-8.

55. Hertzog MJ. Protections of tenure and academic freedom in the United States. Evolution and Interpretation: Springer International Publishing AG; 2017.

Chapter 15

56. Centers for Medicare & Medicaid Services. NHE Fact Sheet [Available from: https://www.cms.gov/Research-Statistics-Data-and-Systems/Statistics-Trends-and-Reports/NationalHealthExpendData/NHE-Fact-Sheet#:~:text=Historical%20NHE%2C%202021%3A,17%20percent%20of%20total%20NHE].

57. Cass, A. The 10 highest paid CEOs at publicly traded health insurance companies [Available from: https://www. beckerspayer.com/payer/the-10-highest-paid-ceos-at-publicly-traded-health-insurance-companies.html.]

58. Summary of the Affordable Care Act [Available from: https://www.kff.org/health-reform/fact-sheet/summary-of-the-affordable-care-act/].

Chapter 16

59. Centers for Medicare & Medicaid Service. Medicare ad Medicaid Helath Information Technology: Title IV of the American Recovery and Reinvestment Act [Available from: https://www.cms.gov/newsroom/fact-sheets/medicare-and-medicaid-health-information-technology-title-iv-american-recovery-and-reinvestment-act.]

60. Harnett K. Female clinicans spend more time with patients and earn less because of it, study shows [Available from: https://www.modernhealthcare.com/compensation/female-clinicians-spend-more-time-patients-and-earn-less-because-it-study-shows].

61. Definitive Healthcare. 10 most common inpatient EHR systems by market share [Available from: https://www.definitivehc.com/blog/most-common-inpatient-ehr-systems.]

62. Medical Economics. Physicians choose their top 7 EHR systems for 2020 [Available from: https://www.medicaleconomics.com/view/physicians-choose-their-top-7-ehr-systems-2019?page=3.]

63. Berg S. Physician burnout: Which medical specialties feel the most stress. AMA Physician Health. 2020.

64. Patel RS, Bachu R, Adikey A, Malik M, Shah M. Factors related to physician burnout and its consequences: A review. Behav Sci (Basel). 2018;8(11).

65. Shen S. *Man's 4th Best Hospital*: Penguin Randome House; 2019.

66. Jabr F. Why the brain prefers paper. Sci Am. 2013;309(5):48-53.

67. Derolf AR, Kristinsson SY, Andersson TM, Landgren O, Dickman PW, Bjorkholm M. Improved patient survival for acute myeloid leukemia: a population-based study of 9729 patients diagnosed in Sweden between 1973 and 2005. Blood. 2009;113(16):3666-72.

68. Summary of the Affordable Care Act [Available from: https://www.kff.org/health-reform/fact-sheet/summary-of-the-affordable-care-act/].

69. Moise KJ, Jr., Rodkey LS, Yared M, Hudon L, Saade G, Dorman K, et al. An animal model for hemolytic disease of the fetus or newborn in New Zealand white and New Zealand red rabbits: newborn effects. Am J Obstet Gynecol. 1998;179(5):1353-8.

Chapter 17

70. Institue of Medicine . Resident Duty Hours. Washington, D.C.: National Academic Press; 2009.

71. Institue of Medicine . Resident Duty Hours. Washington, D.C.: National Academic Press; 2009.

72. Romano PS, Volpp K. The ACGME's 2011 changes to resident duty hours: are they an unfunded mandate on teaching hospitals? J Gen Intern Med. 2012;27(2):136-8.

73. Commitee on Interns and Residents. New ACGME guidelines: Returning to 28-hour on-call shifts [Available from: https://www.cirseiu.org/acgmeresponse/].

74. Institue of Medicine . Resident Duty Hours. Washington, D.C.: National Academic Press; 2009.

75. Williamson AM, Feyer AM. Moderate sleep deprivation produces impairments in cognitive and motor performance equivalent to legally prescribed levels of alcohol intoxication. Occup Environ Med. 2000;57(10):649-55.

76. Bilimoria KY, Chung JW, Hedges LV, Dahlke AR, Love R, Cohen ME, et al. Development of the flexibility in duty hour Rrquirements for surgical trainees (FIRST) trial protocol: A national cluster-randomized trial of resident duty hour policies. JAMA Surg. 2016;151(3):273-81.

77. Basner M, Asch DA, Shea JA, Bellini LM, Carlin M, Ecker AJ, et al. Sleep and alertness in a duty-hour flexibility trial in Internal Medicine. N Engl J Med. 2019;380(10):915-23.

78. National Insitutes of Health. Budget [Available from: https://www.nih.gov/about-nih/what-we-do/budge]t.

79. U.S. News. Find the best medical schools [Available from: https://www.usnews.com/best-graduate-schools/top-medical-schools].

80. Snowden JM, Tilden EL, Snyder J, Quigley B, Caughey AB, Cheng YW. Planned out-of-hospital birth and birth outcomes. N Engl J Med. 2015;373(27):2642-53.

Chapter 18

81. Senat MV, Deprest J, Boulvain M, Paupe A, Winer N, Ville Y. Endoscopic laser surgery versus serial amnioreduction for severe twin-to-twin transfusion syndrome. N Engl J Med. 2004;351(2):136-44.

82. Robinson JV. The "Topping out" traditions of the high-steel ironworkers. W Folore. 2001;60:243-62.

83. Dyer O. Leading US cancer researcher failed to disclose industry ties in dozens of articles. BMJ. 2018;362:k3868.

84. The physician payments Sunshine Act [Available from: https://www.healthaffairs.org/do/10.1377/hpb20141002.272302/full/].

85. Adzick NS, Thom EA, Spong CY, Brock JW, 3rd, Burrows PK, Johnson MP, et al. A randomized trial of prenatal versus postnatal repair of myelomeningocele. N Engl J Med. 2011;364(11):993-1004.

86. Faddick CM. Health care fraud and abuse: new weapons, new penalties, and new fears for providers created by the Health Insurance Portability and Accountability Act of 1996 ("HIPAA"). Ann Health Law. 1997;6:77-104.

Chapter 19

87. Centers for Disease Control and Prevention. History of 1918 Flu Pandemic [Available from: https://www.cdc.gov/flu/

pandemic-resources/1918-commemoration/1918-pandemic-history.htm].

88. World Health Organization. Global Influenza Surveillance and Response System (GISRS) [Available from: https://www.who.int/initiatives/global-influenza-surveillance-and-response-system.]

89. Liew SC, Aung T. Sleep deprivation and its association with diseases- a review. Sleep Med. 2021;77:192-204.

90. Fraser W, Usher RH, McLean FH, Bossenberry C, Thomson ME, Kramer MS, et al. Temporal variation in rates of cesarean section for dystocia: does "convenience" play a role? Am J Obstet Gynecol. 1987;156(2):300-4.

91. Landon MB, Leindecker S, Spong CY, Hauth JC, Bloom S, Varner MW, et al. The MFMU Cesarean Registry: factors affecting the success of trial of labor after previous cesarean delivery. Am J Obstet Gynecol. 2005;193(3 Pt 2):1016-23.

92. Wachter RM, Goldman L. The emerging role of "hospitalists" in the American health care system. N Engl J Med. 1996;335(7):514-7.

93. Maruyama A, Kokuzawa A, Yamauchi Y, Kirino Y, Nagai H, Inoue Y, et al. Clinical features of elderly-onset Adult-onset Still's disease. Mod Rheumatol. 2021;31(4):862-8.

Chapter 20

94. Hesketh PJ, Kris MG, Basch E, Bohlke K, Barbour SY, Clark-Snow RA, et al. Antiemetics: American Society of Clinical Oncology Clinical Practice Guideline Update. J Clin Oncol. 2017;35(28):3240-61.

95. U.S. News Best Hospitals [Available from: https://health. usnews.com/best-hospitals].

96. Statista. Advertising spending in the hospitals industry in the United States from 2020 to 2021 [Available from: https:// www.statista.com/statistics/470699/hospitals-industry- ad-spend-usa/#:~:text=In%20a%20survey%20of%20 representatives,amounted%20to%204.6%20million%20 dollars].

97. Will you live to see 100? Our children and grandchildren have a better chance of becoming centenarians [Available from: https://www.walesonline.co.uk/news/uk-news/ you-live-see-100-children-23073445.]

98. Frangoul H, Ho TW, Corbacioglu S. CRISPR-Cas9 Gene Editing for sickle cell Ddsease and beta-thalassemia. N Engl J Med. 2021;384(23):e91.